FUNDAMENTALS OF PHYSICIAN PRACTICE MANAGEMENT

FUNDAMENTALS OF PHYSICIAN PRACTICE MANAGEMENT

Frederick J. Wenzel
Jane M. Wenzel

Health Administration Press, Chicago, IL
AUPHA Press, Washington, DC

AUPHA
HAP

Your board, staff, or clients may also benefit from this book's insight. For more information on quantity discounts, contact the Health Administration Press Marketing Manager at (312) 424-9470.

09   08   07   06   05   5   4   3   2   1

Library of Congress Cataloging-in-Publication Data

Fundamentals of physician practice management / Frederick J. Wenzel and Jane M. Wenzel, editors.
   p. cm.
   Includes bibliographical references and index.
   ISBN-10: 1-56793-246-0
   ISBN-13: 978-1-56793-246-1
   1. Medicine—Practice. 2. Medical offices—Management. 3. Financial Management. I. Wenzel, Frederick J. II. Wenzel, Jane M.

   R728.F84 2005
   610'.68—dc22

2005050377

The paper used in this publication meets the minimum requirements of American National Standard for Information Sciences—Permanence of Paper for Printed Library Materials, ANSI Z39.48-1984. ∞™

Acquisitions editor: Audrey Kaufman; Project manager: Melissa Rompesky; Cover designer: Trisha Lartz; Layout editor: Amanda Karvelaitis

Health Administration Press
A division of the Foundation
   of the American College of
   Healthcare Executives
One North Franklin Street
Suite 1700
Chicago, IL 60606
(312) 424-2800

Association of University Programs
   in Health Administration
2000 N. 14th Street
Suite 780
Arlington, VA 22201
(703) 894-0940

CONTENTS IN BRIEF

DETAILED CONTENTS

LIST OF FIGURES AND TABLES

FOREWORD

Wenzel and colleagues cover the spectrum of key topics in physician practice management and provide the historical run-up to contemporary physician management practice, ending with a fascinating set of speculations on the future of this form of healthcare management.

The new text could not be better timed. As highly controlled forms of managed care recede in an increasingly market-driven environment, the management and leadership of autonomous physician practices within a context of multiple payers and stakeholders increases in importance.

Chapter 1 provides a brief but potent history of medical group practice, a history that nicely informs the reader as to how and why medical group practice evolved in the way that it did. A key and often overlooked fact is that medical group practice was at first a largely rural American phenomenon, a pattern that surely reinforced the stature of the physician as captain of the ship, a phenomenon with major implications addressed in Chapter 2. The emphasis of rural location on independence, autonomy, and work ethic has penetrated the medical group practice movement and is a critical feature of this form of medical care delivery organization; it must be well understood by anyone wishing to enter into group practice administration.

The authors clearly depict the different managerial roles and responsibilities of the key players in medical group practice and discuss different forms of leadership. An extremely helpful section on common problems faced by physician groups helps the reader understand the pluses and minuses of different leadership structures and is one of the more valuable portions of the entire text.

In the several business and legal models available to physician practices it is the role of the management team to decide which balance between tax advantage and personal liability is to be struck, and the authors adroitly present the advantages and disadvantages of each organizational-corporate approach. The ever-sticky issues of professional liability, antitrust, and compliance are deftly discussed, again in a pithy and accessible format. Finally the all-important question of organization culture is posed; the authors note its critical nature when they write that an organization's culture keeps it on an even keel. The positive and negative forces that flow from culture—inertia versus needed change—are explained.

Chapter 4, which presents strategic planning and marketing, is notable for its precise summary of the principal components of these two management activities and its application to physician practice management. Following this is a treatment of accounting and financial control systems, activities that both are affected by and affect the organization's ability to market and plan strategically. This section, too, is succinctly presented and aptly applied to the physician practice setting. Special attention is paid to the processes of accurate coding, application of fee schedules for reimbursement, and budgeting.

Chapter 6 moves the subject matter to the key issue of physician staffing and management, precisely the area that makes the management of physician practices so special and idiosyncratic. This excellent chapter provides a comprehensive review of what plan administrators must know about planning, recruitment, performance evaluation, compensation and benefits, as well as retention. Wenzel and colleagues then present the subject of information systems in a way that integrates much of the earlier material in the book, as the essence of modern management is timely, accurate, and useful information in all the functional areas of a practice plan. The myriad uses of information systems are clearly laid out for the reader.

Next the book moves to the back office—where the business operations occur, the brains of the entire management effort. Chapter 9 considers the next logical subject: activities that relate to quality, risk management, and the special case of managed care. A solid introduction to the contemporary quality movement is followed by a discussion of how quality and risk management intersect and mutually support each other. The special challenges of administering physician practices in a managed care context close out the section.

The thrust of Chapter 10 is the complicated and challenging issue of physician-hospital relationships, perhaps the most fraught subject that any physician practice manager must deal with in the early twenty-first century. The role of the law in regulating the relationship between physician practices and the hospitals to which they admit their patients is explained in a transparent fashion, not an easy task given the complexity of the contemporary situation. A helpful section on what works caps this important chapter.

The final chapter devotes itself to the future and gives readers glimpses into this murky area through the lens of prominent observers of the physician practice management scene. Issues of cost, quality, automation, and integration repeatedly surface as poles around which change in practice settings will revolve. The authors speculate on the likelihood that various current forms of physician practices will endure and prevail in the coming years. It is fascinating reading that will surely provide much food for debate and investigation.

This is a superb introduction to the quickly changing and challenging world of physician practice management. Readers will have a solid foundation of all the activities that encompass the managerial world in this sector of healthcare delivery. They will be well-prepared for their next steps in the journey toward excellence and leadership in providing the population with accessible and affordable care with a cost-quality ratio that enhances value to all stakeholders—patients, physicians, insurers, vendors, hospitals, and the administrators themselves.

—Stephen S. Mick, PhD, CHE
Arthur Graham Glasgow Professor and Chair
Department of Health Administration
Virginia Commonwealth University

PREFACE

The academic community has shown increasing interest in group practices and the ambulatory care environment as these entities have begun to play a more central role in the healthcare system and the delivery of healthcare services. Many of the graduate programs in healthcare administration began as hospital-oriented degrees but have made a gradual change to a more systems-oriented approach that includes other organizations, especially group practices. The curricula in most undergraduate and graduate programs in health administration have increased in breadth to cover most provider and supply-chain organizations. Group practices have become a new area of emphasis. Few texts are available that make the transition from the core healthcare administration disciplines to the more specialty-oriented aspects of a group practice. Providing a mechanism for making that transition is a primary purpose of this book.

The book is designed to meet the needs of those programs that offer a group practice course as an elective as well as those that incorporate group practice issues into the regular curriculum. This text will also be useful for the professional working in the group practice arena who wishes to gain a broader knowledge of the special issues facing these organizations. It will be especially helpful to those managers who come to a group practice without prior experience in the area.

The book is organized to be used to teach a full-semester course on group practice fundamentals. Each chapter begins with learning objectives and a Case in Point that describes a true-to-life experience to provide a context for the student to understand the information in the chapter. At the end of each chapter are questions that cover the information in that chapter and can be used as discussion points.

The history of the development of group practice is described in Chapter 1 and includes examples of the founding of several large multispecialty practices as well as the discussion of the major professional associations that represent group practices. The four organizations that focus their activities on group practice are the Medical Group Management Association (MGMA), American College of Medical Practice Executives (ACMPE),

American Medical Group Association (AMGA), and American College of Physician Executives (ACPE). These organizations have long histories and continue to make important contributions to the development of the group practice concept. Chapter 2 discusses the leadership and management of medical groups both large and small. All practices, whether they function as part of an integrated system or a freestanding organization, must have an understanding of this evolving area. Members of the senior leadership and management team are defined in terms of their relationships.

Chapter 3 deals with organizational issues, including the different structures within which group practices operate and some of the special legal considerations of group practices. The chapter also includes a discussion of the culture of the organization, which must be understood along with the conflicts frequently found in professional organizations.

Chapter 4 considers planning from the perspectives of strategic and market positioning of the group practice. The principle that, to be effective, strategic and marketing planning should be performed in concert serves as the foundation for the discussion. Special emphasis is placed on the clinician's view of marketing. Chapter 5 deals with the financial and accounting principles peculiar to group practices, with emphasis on reimbursement, financial statements, and compensation for physicians. Chapter 6 considers human resources and staffing issues in group practices; these issues are not unlike those in other healthcare institutions in certain ways, but some differences must be observed.

Chapters 7 and 8 are companion chapters dealing with information systems and the operational issues facing group practices. Information systems have become the central nervous systems of physician organizations just as they have with other healthcare organizations. However, some data and management information issues are unique to group practices, especially issues related to the adoption of automated systems by professionals. The operation of day-to-day practice is also different than in the hospital setting, and an understanding of the need for "right now" approaches to operational issues is important.

Chapter 9 deals with three closely interrelated issues: quality, risk, and managed care. Although we do not provide a comprehensive discussion of these topics, the chapter contains sufficient information to provide the student with a good background on the importance of quality assessment and improvement and the risks encountered in group practices. Managed care has become a way of life for physician organizations, and an understanding of managed care principles and their relation to risk and quality is key.

Chapter 10 contains a most important discussion of physician-hospital relationships and how they have evolved over the past 10 to 15 years. In this chapter the student will find emphasis on the importance of professionals and hospitals working together for the future success of the healthcare delivery system. Despite an often significant competition between the two groups, they must move to cooperation if they are to be successful. The future of group practice is discussed in Chapter 11 in light of the many issues and complexities facing the healthcare system. The primary role that group practices will play as the system becomes more integrated is considered from the perspective that the group practice will serve as the principle building block of the system.

This book provides solid background on the fundamentals of group practice and the ambulatory care environment. Rather than supplant the core courses traditionally taught in either undergraduate or graduate health administration programs, it is meant to build on them and reinforce and broaden the perspective of students. The book will also have value for managers entering group practice organizations who have not had experience in that area. This is especially true for managers who move from the hospital to the group practice setting. Managing in a group practice is different from managing in a hospital, and a successful manager must understand the physician culture and the uniqueness of the professional organization.

ACKNOWLEDGMENTS

The authors are indebted to Audrey Kaufman and Melissa Rompesky, who worked tirelessly on this project, and to our spouses, Mary Ann Wenzel, Terri Ryan Mitlyng, Jeanne White, and Tim Nelson, whose patience and encouragement made it all possible. We are also grateful to our children, friends, and employers for their support. The authors would also like to recognize Stephen Mick for his insightful foreword as well as the MGMA experts Dick Hansen, Bob Bohlmann, Darrell Schryver, and Hobie Collins for their view of the future of a group practice.

HISTORICAL DEVELOPMENTS IN MEDICAL GROUP PRACTICE

Frederick J. Wenzel

Learning Objectives

This chapter will enable the reader to

- understand the historic developments leading to modern group practices;
- acquire a working knowledge of the factors leading to medical group formation;
- develop a sense of how the past and present will affect the group practice of the future;
- understand the different forms group practices have adopted and the importance of specialization; and
- understand the role and influence of professional organizations on the growth of a group practice.

Chapter Purpose

This chapter outlines the historical developments related to group practices. While it is difficult to trace the early history in a precise fashion, milestones have been identified. The chapter examines the primary drivers as well as the barriers to the development of physician groups. Also discussed is the group practice of the future. The role of professional organizations and societies founded to support group practices is also included. The historical development of leadership and management in physician organizations is traced to provide a foundation for later chapters on that topic. The histories of several pioneer group practices are described in sufficient detail so the reader will be able to understand when, how, and why they started. These groups continue to be important contributors to the group practice movement.

Case in Point

Doctor Johnson was interviewing a prospective physician who was interested in locating in the area where Dr. Johnson was medical director of a multispecialty clinic. The physician asked Dr. Johnson a number of questions about group practice, especially regarding when they originated and what some of the advantages of joining a group practice were. Dr. Johnson thought for a moment and then responded. "It is difficult to identify the exact origin of group practices, but their appearance can be traced to the early part of the last century." The discussion continued for some time, and then Dr. Johnson said: "I have two questions for you. The first is, 'Why are you interested in practicing in a group?' The second is, 'What do you think the advantages and disadvantages might be in becoming a member of a group where, as some have suggested, you might lose some of your autonomy?'" The discussion that followed was very interesting and insightful. How would you have answered?

Early History

Group Practice Defined

> Medical group practice: an original American phenomenon, largely inspired by the first major group, the Mayo Clinic; its appearance coincided with specialization in medicine and much of the early growth was fed by the experience of American physicians who served in the American expeditionary Force during World War I (Madison 1990, p. 52).

Identifying the origin and tracing the history of the group practice of medicine presents a significant challenge. It is difficult to find an exact date or even a series of dates identifying the birth of this important aspect of the healthcare delivery system. More has been written about the histories of the professional organizations that evolved in support of group practice (Medical Group Management Association [MGMA], American College of Medical Practice Executives [ACMPE], American Medical Group Association [AMGA], and American College of Physician Executives [ACPE]). Thus, some of the detail outlined in this chapter has been taken from the history of these associations' activities.

The first and perhaps only comprehensive history of ambulatory care was written by Donald Madison in 1990. Madison traced the origin and development of the dispensary as a forerunner to the delivery of care in the outpatient setting. Typically these care facilities were associated with hospitals, but eventually they evolved into freestanding outpatient care organizations. Schneck (2004) traced the roots of group practice back to the late nineteenth century. A number of factors contributed to the emergence of group practice. The most often cited reasons were the new age of scientific advances and the need for specialization to deal with developments in the delivery of healthcare. Thus specialization and the "new technology" became drivers as physicians began to collaborate and form groups with mutual interests. Despite later focus on quality and cost, their role during the early days of group practice formation is uncertain. The second factor driving the rise of group practice models, unusual as it may sound, was the development of full-time medical school faculties, which is discussed later in this chapter.

There have been a variety of definitions of group practice. The current definition of medical group practice adopted by the American Medical Association (AMA) is, "the provision of health care services by a group of at least three licensed physicians engaged in a formally organized and legally recognized entity: sharing equipment, facilities, common records, and personnel involved in both patient care and business management" (Havlicek 1984, p. 1). This suggests a medical group is defined by organizational characteristics rather than function. The Center for Research in Ambulatory Health Care Administration of MGMA (American Group Practice Association, et al. 1978) proposed that "group medical practice is a process, not a form of organization." A number of significant arguments support that position. In 1931, Rorem (p. 6) suggested:

> Group medical practice characterizes the full time activities of many physicians employed by government agencies, business corporations, medical schools, hospitals and other agencies. But the most widespread and significant form of group medical practice is a voluntary association of private practitioners who form partnerships or otherwise organize with the purpose of assuming joint responsibility for care of patients and for income distribution.

Since the AMA was founded as a professional society of solo practitioners, its members expressed concern about the development of group practice. This apprehension related principally to the perceived loss of focus on the objectives of the individual physician as compared with the objectives of the group. Group practice was seen as a socialistic approach to the practice of medicine, which would intrude on the physician-patient relationship. The AMA also considered a number of other issues to be of concern, including the employer-employee relationship of group practice physicians; prepayment of medical services, which might threaten the integrity of the physician-patient relationship; and the involvement by group practices in consumer-controlled healthcare cooperatives. The rationale for the opposition to these organizations, which represented the clients, was that they would dictate physicians' income and working conditions (MGMA 1976). A number of intense discussions among the professionals involved in these issues took place, especially in the early part of the last century.

More recently, however, the AMA has altered its position and has created within its organizational structure a group practice committee that communicates with the body of the organization about the status of and issues facing group practices. While there remain remnants of resistance within the AMA, the group practice model is generally accepted. In fact, a significant portion of the membership of the AMA is made up of group practice physicians.

Factors Influencing the Growth of Group Practice

A variety of other factors influenced the development of group practice.

Need for Medical Care in Rural America

Providing medical care to address the needs of rural populations has always been a challenge in this country. Early in the last century a number of physician groups formed to meet that need. An AMA survey (MGMA 1976) reported that half of the medical groups established by 1933 were in cities with populations of fewer than 25,000 people; two thirds were in cities of fewer than 50,000. Only 4 percent served larger cities with populations of more than 500,000 people.

World War II

World War II also had a significant impact on not only the development of new group practices but the growth of existing practices as well. The GI Bill encouraged young men to enter college, and many of these students subsequently made their way to medical school. There was a significant increase in the number of group practices beginning in the early 1950s as a direct result of this phenomenon.

Development of Healthcare Financing Alternatives

Another phenomenon that stimulated the formation of group practices was the development of alternative financing mechanisms to cover the cost of medical care. This movement led to the development of the health maintenance organization (HMO), which was formalized through federal legislation in the early 1970s. It was the Kaiser organization that first developed the concept of prepayment for medical services, which eventually led to the founding of the Kaiser Permanente Medical Group in 1933 (Kaiser Permanente 2003). This movement was followed by the development of staff model cooperatives around the country, some of which are still in existence today. They are true cooperatives. The patients or enrollees are the owners of the organization, and they contract with individual physicians to staff the cooperative and provide medical services. These cooperatives were quite troublesome for the AMA because of the ownership issue.

While most group practices formed during the last century were for-profit organizations, there has been a significant move during the last 30 years toward the development of not-for-profit 501(c)(3) organizations for large multispecialty groups. It is also interesting to note that most academic health centers were also tax-exempt organizations, and in the past ten years many have evolved into the foundation model. In the past many medical school departments operated as independent 501(c)(3) organizations. However, with the increasing complexity in legal and compliance issues as well as the economic aspects of practice, there was a move in the 1990s to form a single not-for-profit organization—often called a foundation, a word taken from the IRS code—under which the departmental organizations fall. Some states, such as California, prohibit the corporate practice of medicine; in these areas "foundations for medical care" were developed as the organizational model for group practices. Organizationally they look much like the 501(c)(3)s described above.

Thus group practices grew rapidly in the latter in part of the twentieth century, and that growth continues through the opening decade of the twenty-first century. By 1998 there were some 16,000 groups in the United States, and that number has grown in the past five years to nearly 20,000. The growth in the number of groups is primarily related to single-specialty organizations, whereas the growth in the total number of physicians is for the most part in multispecialty practice organizations. Over the years some transformation of single-specialty practices into multispecialty practices has occurred. The driver in these cases is the broadening of the delivery process and the perceived need for a group of family physicians to add other specialties such as pediatrics, obstetrics, or general surgery.

Group Practice Models

Group practice has two principal forms, single specialty and multispecialty. As the name implies, single-specialty groups focus on a single aspect of medicine such as general surgery, family practice, orthopedics, internal medicine, cardiology, urology, or a host of other specialties and subspecialties. Multispecialty groups have nearly all of the specialties and subspecialties of medicine and surgery represented. Most of these organizations have a highly integrated structure. Management teams made up of both physicians and administrators deal with the issues related to governance, leadership, and management. More and more multispecialty and large single-specialty groups are finding it necessary to establish highly refined corporate structures to deal with the complexities of the financial and regulatory systems that have evolved around the healthcare system and medical practice.

The Pioneers

This same period heralded the emergence of significant developments in the sophistication of the delivery of ambulatory care and the group practice of medicine. The history of group practice might best be described by relating the history of several groups and why and how they started.

The Mayo Clinic

The Mayo Clinic in Rochester, Minnesota, was founded by the "Brothers Mayo–William and Charles." Their vision included the development of specialization and subspecialization of medical care based on the complexity of a rapidly growing healthcare system. The Mayos believed physicians could practice better medicine in a collegial group environment than on an individual basis, and that the quality of service to patients would be enhanced in this kind of environment. In 1883 a devastating tornado struck Rochester, causing many casualties. In response the doctors Mayo teamed up with the Sisters of St. Francis and formed a relationship that lasted for more than 90 years. The Mayo Clinic was founded in the late 1880s, when the two brothers joined their father in practice in Rochester. They were joined later by Drs. Augustus Stinchfield (1892), Christopher Graham (1895), Milvin Millet (1898), and Henry Plummer (1901). Dr. Louis Wilson was added to the group in 1905 to develop the laboratories. When the business of the clinic became increasingly complicated the doctors asked local banker Harry J. Harwick to join the organization. He turned out to be a significant asset and is widely recognized as the first formal group practice administrator. Harwick remained with the group for many years (Mayo Foundation for Medical Education and Research 2004), and he became one of the founders of MGMA.

The Mayo Clinic has grown substantially since its founding. This growth was especially remarkable near the end of the last century, when sites were developed in Scottsdale, Arizona; Jacksonville, Florida; and throughout Minnesota and Wisconsin. At the same time the group acquired the two hospitals in Rochester, developed a medical school, and continued its significant and ever-growing medical research program. In 2004 the system cared for 513,000 unique patients (defined as one patient, regardless of how many times he is seen in a year) and had 2,271,484 total outpatient visits. The Mayo Foundation employs 47,878 full- and part-time staff members, with a total of more than 2,968 physicians and scientists. The Mayo Clinic is the most recognized healthcare organization in the country, if not in the entire world (Mayo Foundation for Medical Education and Research 2003).

Scott & White Memorial

On October 1, 1890 Dr. Arthur C. Scott, Sr., began his career at the Santa Fe Hospital in Temple, Texas. Shortly thereafter he held a competitive examination for those who applied for the vacant post of Santa Fe Hospital house surgeon. Dr. Raleigh R. White, Jr., of Cameron, Texas, scored the highest on the exam and was hired. These physicians entered into a full partnership in December of 1887. In 1904 the doctors opened their own hospital, the Temple Sanitarium, and later that year purchased and converted an abandoned convent for use as a permanent hospital. That structure became the nucleus of a campus that today has 31 buildings scattered over five city blocks. The organization includes the Scott & White Memorial Hospital and the Scott, Sherwood & Brindley Foundation (Scott & White 2004a).

Thus began a clinic-based system staffed by physicians who later developed their own hospital, clinic, medical school relationship, and research program. In 1933 the Scott & White Clinic became the first American College of Surgeons–approved cancer treatment center in Texas.

The Scott & White Clinic and Hospital, with the Scott & White Health Plan, now constitutes one of the largest multispecialty group practices in the United States. A model of integrated halthcare, Scott and White (2004b) consists of a 500 plus physician clinic, a 486 bed hospital, and a health plan that covers more than 167,000 central Texans.

The Marshfield Clinic

The Marshfield Clinic in Marshfield, Wisconsin, was founded in 1916 by Dr. K. W. Doege and five enterprising physicians who believed the best way to practice was in a group where they could share knowledge, facilities, and services. The group was located in rural central Wisconsin, an important rail center for lumbering at the time. The Marshfield Clinic teamed up with the Sisters of the Sorrowful Mother, who had founded St. Joseph's Hospital just before the turn of the century. The group, which remains freestanding, has grown rapidly and today has 727 physicians and 5,815 staff members and has clinics in 48 communities in central and northern Wisconsin. It has its own insurance plan, Security Health Plan, which was started in the early 1970s as one of Wisconsin's first HMOs. The plan began as a partnership between BlueCross and St. Joseph's Hospital and was later purchased by the clinic in 1986. The Marshfield Clinic has strong teaching and research programs (Marshfield Clinic 2005).

The Carle Clinic

The Carle Clinic was founded in the 1920s by Drs. J. C. Thomas and Hugh L. Davison. These two young physicians, who trained at the Mayo Clinic, believed they could transfer the Mayo concept of multispecialty group medical practice to east central Illinois. They believed patients in rural areas should have access to advanced medicine near their homes. The Carle Clinic is associated with the Carle Foundation Hospital, a 300-bed tertiary care unit that houses a level 1 trauma center and a center for the treatment of cancer. The clinic has more than 300 physicians in a multispecialty practice, with a network of branch clinics throughout the region (Carle Clinic Association and Carle Foundation Hospital 2003).

Virginia Mason Medical Center

Virginia Mason Medical Center, located in metropolitan Seattle, was established in 1920 as an 80-bed hospital with six physician offices. The founders' vision was to provide a single place where patients could receive comprehensive medical care, a one-stop shop for virtually any medical problem. Today the medical center houses a multispecialty group practice of more than 390 physicians who offer both primary and specialized care. The center also has a regional network of neighborhood clinics, an internationally recognized research institute, and a philanthropic foundation (Virginia Mason Medical Center 2004).

The Fargo Clinic

The Fargo Clinic, located in Fargo, North Dakota, and now part of the MeritCare Health System, opened its doors in 1921. The founders believed that physicians practicing as a group could provide primary and specialized care to patients as a team, offering better quality and more cost-efficient care. The founders of the clinic were Drs. Sand, Cronnes, and Oftedahl. Dr. Sands envisioned creating a small-scale Mayo Clinic on the prairies of North Dakota (MeritCare Health System 2005).

The Geisinger Clinic

The Geisinger Clinic of Danville, Pennsylvania, was founded by Dr. Harold L. Foss in 1915. Foss trained with Drs. William and Charles Mayo at the Mayo Clinic and, like other Mayo-trained physicians, dreamed of establishing a similar clinic in his region. The clinic is associated with a hospital built by Abigail Geisinger in 1885 (Geisinger Health System 2003).

This brief account of the development of these groups in various parts of the United States provides a sense of the evolution of group practice and its founders' ideals. Undoubtedly many other clinic groups founded in the nineteenth and twentieth centuries could also be noted; however, the clinics described above are especially notable because they have survived and continue to thrive despite the challenges of the current healthcare climate.

The Academic Medical Center

Academic health centers and medical school faculty physician groups have evolved especially over the past 10 to 15 years. These centers associated with medical schools have a strong departmental orientation with significant resistance to a more corporate central structure, unlike most medical care systems, which have now adopted a corporate structure to deal with the complexities of both the delivery of care and administration. A number of academic health centers have combined their departments into a multispecialty group foundation, described earlier. The foundation serves as the corporate structure and performs billing, collecting, and management functions. The foundation also serves as a vehicle for quality assurance programs, community service, and the development of compensation systems. The departmental model of the medical school provides significant autonomy from both the service and administrative perspectives. The financial responsibility is part of the departmental structure, and the chair has a great deal of authority. The change to a foundation model has caused conflict because of the cultural shift and the perceived appearance of a loss of power by the department and its chair.

It will be important to follow the evolution of these systems, which are sure to mature rapidly as cost pressures and regulation complexities continue to escalate. The deans of most medical schools have been supportive of the development of the foundation model, which, although separate, is a primary contributor to the educational mission of the medical school. It is not clear at this point what senior university officials think about this evolution, but it appears most are supportive. In the future academic health centers will likely resemble the freestanding multispecialty clinics described earlier in this chapter.

Medical Group Practice Associations

The principal group practice associations are MGMA, ACMPE, AMGA, and ACPE. They were formed to provide member services to those individuals engaged in leadership and management of group practices and related organizations. They provide education, service, and research and lobby on behalf of their members. While having a common interest, each organization has a special emphasis.

Medical Group Management Association (MGMA)
The founding concept of individuals and organizations working together and sharing knowledge was unveiled in 1926 in Madison, Wisconsin, when a group of 22 managers representing 14 clinics met to discuss issues of mutual interest. They formed MGMA to accomplish their goals. The concept was obviously a good one because by 1932 the association was home to about 300 medical groups. The association has grown rapidly and today has more than 19,500 members in 11,500 organizations that represent 240,000 physicians (MGMA 2005).

Madison (1990, p. 43) stated,

> The roots of MGMA were planted in one tradition.... And the association still reflects primarily the interests of the private clinic...but MGMA over the years borrowed methods from and grew with members from every tradition until it transcended the boundaries and stands now as the common denominator of today's group practice.

ACMPE was born out of MGMA's interest in education and the certification of its members. Its fellows can be found in many healthcare organizations around the country. The two associations host an annual meeting each year, attracting nearly 5,000 participants.

American Medical Group Association (AMGA)

AMGA, formerly the American Group Practice Association (AGPA), was founded in 1949 as the American Association of Medical Clinics (AAMC). The association has both group and individual members. According to AMGA's (2004) history,

> The American Medical Group Association (AMGA) represents medical groups, including some of the nation's largest, most prestigious integrated healthcare delivery systems. AMGA advocates for the multispecialty medical group model of healthcare delivery and for the patients served by medical groups through innovation and informaton sharing, benchmarking, leadership development, and continuous striving to improve patient care. The members of AMGA deliver healthcare to more than 50 million patients in 42 states, including 15 million capitated lives. Headquartered in Alexandria, Virginia, AMGA is the strategic partner for medical groups providing a comprehensive package of benefits, including political advocacy, educational and networking programs and publications, benchmarking data services, and financial and operations assistance.

American College of Physician Executives (ACPE)

ACPE was founded in 1975 to promote leadership and management education for physicians. The organization, located in Tampa, Florida, conducts many different kinds of educational seminars and has relationships with degree-granting universities. In addition the association awards certificates to its members who attain specific educational goals. The organization, made up of individual physicians, grew from 5,700 in 1990 to 14,000 in 2004.

Evolution of Group Practice Governance and Management

As group practices evolve there is a continuing need to develop effective governance and management systems. This topic is discussed in greater detail in subsequent chapters.

With the small physician group, governance and management are typically informal processes. Not infrequently the group will be led by a physician who was a founder or who has agreed to accept the position without election. The manager may well be someone who has little background in management but has been an outstanding nurse or staff member. The position of manager may also be filled by the individual responsible for the billing process. As the group begins to grow and mature it is necessary to have a group of physicians responsible for the governance of the organization and someone with training to deal with the management responsibilities. This is a difficult transition for most groups. Often the physician leader is the founder of the group and has an informal management style under which it may be difficult to promote direction and vision for the organization.

The next phase of growth and development is characterized by a process in which a physician president is elected from the group at large. This happens in groups having between 25 and 75 physicians. The group also selects a manager who has had some training and experience with group practices. A group of this size will almost always have a board of directors or executive committee that becomes part of its formal governance structure.

In the next stage of development the clinic will likely have not only a president, but also a medical director who is responsible for the medical affairs of the organization and issues related to quality. The manager or administrator will have a degree in a related area. Today individuals with masters degrees are being retained for these positions. Groups in this category generally have from 75 to 150 physicians. Groups of 150 physicians or more have an increasing need for governance, leadership, and management. They will have a formal board of directors, elected on a periodic basis. The management will expand to include an executive administrator, medical director, general counsel, chief financial officer, director of human resources, manager of clinical services, information systems director, and director of marketing and communications. Group practices of substantial size have structures that look much like those of a traditional hospital.

Group Practice Benefits

There are a number of factors related to the purpose and benefits of group practice, many of which have been cited earlier in this chapter. Schneck (2004) described them well:

- Offer health professionals the opportunity to interact with each other, encouraging them to seek opinions from peers in managing complex health problems
- Benefit the community by serving as the primary source and resource for health information
- Attract new physicians to the community

- Provide complex services on site such as laboratory testing and X-ray and other kinds of imaging and bone density measurements with a high level of quality
- Allow physicians to develop standardized initiatives for quality such as clinical guidelines, accurate coding, documentation, and standardized operations, streamlining care for patients
- Increase patient access through extended office hours, evening and weekend hours, and on-call coverage
- Implement efficiencies in business administration, billing, coding, reimbursement, and quality improvement
- Contain medical costs through economies of scale for staff and supplies, and in the use of technology to provide less expensive services in ambulatory settings
- Give patients a variety of healthcare services with multiple providers in one location
- Provide physicians with a stable lifestyle and offer camaraderie that contributes to their security and satisfaction
- Allow physicians to practice medicine with minimal concern for the day-to-day operations handled by the office staff
- Offer physicians mentoring opportunities. New physicians learn from established physicians; established physicians stay abreast of new knowledge and techniques by affiliation with newly trained physicians

These important factors can best be defined as the collegiality necessary to provide the foundation for group practice culture. Group practice is all about sharing from every perspective. Not all physicians fit into such a model. However, the last two generations of physicians are increasingly interested not only in medical service, but also in the opportunities for research and education found in larger group practices. Group practice offers lifestyle choices related to location, hours, and style of practice, factors important to the current generation of physicians.

According to Casalino et al. (2003), the following factors are important in the organizational development of large medical practices: leverage with health plans, economies of scale, leverage with hospitals, profit from ancillary services, better lifestyle, and quality improvement.

The Future of Group Practice

The barriers to group practice formation are decreasing rapidly. At one time physicians were extremely independent and held the belief that they could do virtually everything better by themselves. Autonomy was seen as an important aspect of the physician-patient relationship. Because of the complexity of the delivery of healthcare services, management of the financial aspects of practice, and significant governmental regulation and intervention, there has been a significant change in how individuals feel about being part of a group. A sense of fierce independence seems to have waned significantly in the last 10 to 25 years.

Barriers do exist, as cited by Casalino et al. (2003): lack of physician cooperation, lack of capital, lack of physician leadership, cost considerations, and primary care–specialist conflicts.

Abundant evidence demonstrates that most residents who complete their training join a group practice of one kind or another. Some migrate toward single-specialty groups, whereas others choose multispecialty groups because of the advantages of practicing with a variety of different specialties. The day of the solo practitioner appears to be on the wane, and in the next ten years virtually all physicians will likely be practicing within either single or multispecialty groups.

As group practices continue to evolve and develop from a cottage industry into a multibillion-dollar-a-year medical business, there will be continuing emphasis on physicians and others developing group practices. It is difficult to say where it will all end, but economists tell us healthcare spending will increase over the next eight to ten years to 17 percent to 18 percent of the gross domestic product, resulting in an expenditure of more than $3.1 trillion.

If there is to be control over the system, one of the ways in which it can be achieved is by working with organizations such as group practices in which the physicians actually control much of the traffic and expenditures. After all, physicians admit patients to hospitals and order virtually all the studies done on patients as well as prescribe treatments and drugs. Thus group practice will have a significant impact on the healthcare of the future.

Summary

The history of group practice is difficult to trace. If one examines the growth and development of some of the larger groups there are a number of lessons that shed light on how these organizations evolved. The story begins in the early part of the twentieth century with a few early starts in the late 1800s. Group practices in general were born out of a vision held by a number of physicians that high-quality care could be delivered most efficiently in the group setting. The initial evolution appears to have been populated principally by multispecialty practices but later there appeared single-specialty groups, which have since enjoyed significant success.

There are a number of barriers to the development of group practices, most of which are related to a strong feeling of professional standards and physician autonomy. To overcome this environment it is necessary that collegiality occupy a strong position in the culture of the organization. In modern times there has been a continuing expansion of the membership in medium-sized and large multispecialty groups. Single-specialty groups have grown both numbers of organizations and membership in those organizations. There are a number of models that can be found in group practices, including corporations, partnerships, foundations, and cooperatives.

Discussion Questions

1. What were some of the driving forces behind the development of the group practice of medicine?
2. What can you say about the evolution of governance in a group practice?
3. What is the rationale for specialization?
4. Why is it important to understand the evolution of a group practice?
5. Why is it important to understand the barriers to group practice formation?

References

American Group Practice Association, American Medical Association, et al. 1978. *Group Practice: Guidelines to Forming or Joining a Medical Group.* Denver: Center for Research in Ambulatory Health Care Administration.

American Medical Group Association. 2004 "Who We Are." [Online information; retrieved 9/9/04.] www.amga.org/WhoWeAre/history_whoWeAre.asp.

Carle Clinic Association and Carle Foundation Hospital. 2003. "About Us." [Online information; retrieved 9/5/04.] www.carle.com/CFH/about/history .com.

Casalino, L. P., K. J. Devers, T. K. Lake, M. Reed, and J. J. Stoddard. 2003. "Benefits of and Barriers to Large Medical Group Practice in the United States." *Archives of Internal Medicine* 163 (16): 1958–64.

Geisinger Health System. 2003. "About Geisinger." [Online information; retrieved 9/5/04.] www.geisinger.org/about/history.shtml.

Havlicek, P. L. 1984. *Medical Groups in the U.S.* Chicago: American Medical Association.

Kaiser Permanente. 2003. "Physicians Team up to Provide Care for Thousands." [Online information; retrieved 2/15/05.] https://newsmedia.kaiser permanente.org/kpweb/historykp/navlinkpage.do?elementId=htmlapp /feature/121historykp/nat_history2.html.xml&repositoryBean=/kp /repositories/ContentRepository.

Madison, D. L. 1990. "Notes on the History of Group Practice: The Tradition of the Dispensary." *Medical Group Management Journal* 37 (5): 52–54, 56–60, 86–93.

Marshfield Clinic. 2005. "About Us." [Online information; retrieved 2/15/05.] www.marshfieldclinic.org/marshfieldclinic/pages/default.aspx?page=about _legacy.

Mayo Foundation for Medical Education and Research. 2003. "2003 Statistics." [Online information; retrieved 9/24/04.] www.mayoclinic.org/about /history.html.

———. 2004. "History." [Online information; retrieved 9/24/04.] www.mayo clinic.org/about/facts.html.

Medical Group Management Association. 1976. *The History of the Medical Group Management Association.* Denver: Medical Group Management Association.

———. 2005. "About Us." [Online information; retrieved 4/25/05.] www.mgma.com/about/.

MeritCare Health System. 2005. "History." [Online information; retrieved 9/5/04.] www.meritcare.com/about/history/1919.asp.

Rorem, C. R. 1931. *Private Group Clinics: The Administrative and Economic Aspects of Group Medical Practice.* Chicago: University of Chicago Press.

Scott & White. 2004a. "Over 100 Years of Excellence." [Online information; retrieved 9/4/04.] www.sw.org/sw/portal/.cmd/SWActionDispatcher /_pagr/107/_pa.107/116/.swaction/org.sw.browse/.swdoc/iwcontent ~public~corpinfo~en_us~html~corpinfo_aboutus_history.jsp/.piid/152 /.ciid/253.

———. 2004b. "Frequently Asked Questions About Scott & White." [Online information; retrieved 2/15/05.] www.sw.org/sw/portal/.cmd/SWAction Dispatcher/_pagr/107/_pa.107/116/.swaction/org.sw.browse/.swdoc /iwcontent~public~corpinfo~en_us~html~corpinfo_faq.jsp/.piid/152/.ciid /253#.

Schneck, L. H. 2004. "Strength in Numbers. Medical Group Practices Fill Vital Niche in U.S. Health Care System." *MGMA Connexion* 4 (1): 34–43.

Virginia Mason Medical Center. 2004. "About Virginia Mason." [Online information; retrieved 9/4/04.] www.virginiamason.org/about/default.htm.

LEADERSHIP AND MANAGEMENT OF PHYSICIAN GROUPS

Joseph W. Mitlyng

Learning Objectives

This chapter will enable the reader to:

- understand the unique characteristics of physician practices and their influence on the leadership and management of the groups;
- understand the definitions, roles, and responsibilities of the leadership and management positions including the president, administrator, and medical director;
- understand the criteria for leadership effectiveness as individuals and members of the leadership team;
- identify ways to evaluate the success of the model that has been adopted to test the effectiveness of the leadership and management team, especially as it relates to the physician-administrator team; and
- assess examples of effective and ineffective ways for the leadership team to handle common issues that arise in the management of physician groups.

Chapter Purpose

This chapter provides an overview and working knowledge of the leadership and management characteristics of physician group practice. Examples of traits of leadership team members are provided, and these individuals' roles and responsibilities are defined. Criteria important to the evaluation of the success of the team are considered. Also addressed are the challenges of leading and managing a group of physicians, an understanding of which will provide the reader with the tools necessary to lead all groups of ambulatory care providers. The decision process necessary for success forms an important foundation for the discussion. Principles are presented as related to hospital-owned as well as independent, freestanding groups owned by their members.

Case in Point

John Williams recently graduated with a masters degree in healthcare administration and has been looking for a position in medical group management. He has no prior experience in working with physicians as a medical group administrator, but he has just been recruited by Community Physicians Group as its first formally trained administrator.

John is meeting with Dr. James Mitchell, the president of the group. Dr. Mitchell says, "John, I am looking forward to working with you. Our previous administrator, Mike Smith, was with us for about 20 years. He was with us through some significant growth, from fewer than 10 physicians to the more than 40 physicians we have today. But it was time for him to retire. When we were smaller, there was plenty of revenue to keep everyone happy. Mike's gruffness—'If I think you need to know something about the details of how the practice is doing financially, I will tell you'—was accepted by those of us who started the group and knew and trusted Mike. But that style is not acceptable to the younger members of the group, and his relationship with them was deteriorating. I hope you and I will be able to develop a leadership and management team that will work well with the members of the group. I would like you to develop a plan for your activities over the next four to eight weeks as you start work here—what you plan to do and how you and I should work together. I expect you have been giving your first steps here some thought. I would like to meet with you the day after tomorrow to go over your plan." What characteristics should John have to be successful?

Characteristics of a Physician Group

Physician groups share many characteristics with other professional groups, but one characteristic, as discussed below, is unique.

Shared Characteristics

Accounting, law, engineering, and other consulting firms have many of the same characteristics as physician groups.

Members of the Group Generate the Revenue Those who provide the core services are often also the owners of the group. In each case junior professionals may not yet be members of the group, but membership is typically some form of professional partnership in which each member is rewarded in proportion to their revenue generated, their other contributions to the clinic, and the overall success of the practice.

Some costs of the practice can be identified at the level of the individual practice, for example, staff who work solely as part of a single practice site or for a single practicing member. Other costs for centralized services, such as computer systems, billing and collections, and organizational accounting, are examples of group costs.

Both Group and Individual Costs Can Be Identified

Developing a client base is a major challenge in any professional services firm. Membership in a respected, successful group provides immediate market recognition and acceptance by existing and potential clients. An individual member may be new to the clinic but still find himself with a busy practice just serving the existing customers of the firm.

Value in Being Part of a Successful Group

Professional service firms have been described as organizations where the major assets walk in during the morning and walk out at night; the major assets of the firm are the skills of the people employed by it. The firm may have a noncompete clause, but such clauses are often difficult to enforce. The customers/clients/patients can still choose where they want to buy their services. Individuals who feel the firm is not serving them well can choose to leave the firm and, alone or with others, set up a competing firm. Ensuring that individuals are well-satisfied with their membership in the firm is a leadership and management priority in a professional services firm.

Individuals Can Establish a Competing Group

Unique Characteristic

One defining characteristic of physician groups is unique: each physician is trained to be the "captain of the ship," with total and final say and accountability for the care provided to his patients. In accounting, law, engineering, and other service firms the work product of individual professionals is subject to review by superiors before it is given to the client. This does not happen in medical care. The physician's care is immediate. He/she gathers and review the patient's information, decides on a course of action, and implements it to care for her patient. The physician is the captain of the ship, legally and professionally responsible for all of the care the patient does and does not receive. The review that does take place occurs when there is time for review, retrospectively. This review can provide support for the decisions made or ideas on what to do differently next time, but it does not change the immediate responsibility the physician had in the care of her patient.

Immediate and complete responsibility for their patients has a profound effect on the expectations and requirements physicians have for the leadership and management of their medical groups. Physicians expect medical group leaders to be immediately responsive to their concerns and to have achieved a high level of competence and performance in their area(s) of responsibility.

Implications of the "Captain of the Ship" Philosophy

The autonomy of the physician in caring for patients requires self-directed staff who can decide how to best support the physician. Physicians expect to be involved in decisions affecting their day-to-day practice. Meeting that expectation results in better physician performance.

Self-directed Staff

Physician groups are organizations in which it seems nobody tells anybody what to do.

- The pace and structure of practice do not allow time for supervisor direction.
- Staff must be self-directed.
- Physicians do not respond well to hierarchical direction.

Performance expectations are established in well-run physician groups. The expectations may be the result of formal discussions and documentation in writing. More often they have been established as a set of implicit understandings of how the practice is to function, which results from the experience of working together. Some examples:

- Dr. Smith is scheduled to take an hour for lunch, but she will always use that time to fit in patients who need to be seen today. She mentioned this morning that she has an outside appointment this noon.
- Dr. Jones will always work in a patient who arrives late; Dr. Kent will generally require the patient to reschedule the visit for another time. Dr. Kent has said he needs to see an established patient, Mrs. Wills, even if she arrives late today.
- There is a need for the doctor who is in the office to admit Mrs. Stone, a patient who requires immediate attention and a cardiology consult.

The office staff who work directly with the physicians and patients must be able to act independently. They must be self-directed and capable of making decisions and acting without the benefit of continuous supervisor guidance. Except in those unusual cases in which the staff member does not know what to do and must ask the supervisor for assistance, there is no time for supervisor direction in a busy office practice.

Individuals who succeed in a self-directed environment do not respond well to top-down, or hierarchical, direction. The environment of a busy practice is sometimes described as "in the heat of battle." Jobs can be challenging, with minute-to-minute decisions. Individual staff members, like the physicians they work with, want to know why a change is being proposed before they agree to make a modification that may add more complexity to what they already see as a complex, challenging job. As an example, staff in a busy office practice will typically respond to a directive such as, "As you room each patient, I want you to make a check mark on this form," with a question: "Why?" The question will be there whether it is stated or not. Answering the why (in a way that makes sense to the staff) is the first step to getting accurate check-mark information.

The top three leadership positions in a medical group and the concept of the physician-administrator team are outlined later in the chapter. These positions are responsible for the overall functioning and strategic direction of the group, but the business of the business occurs each day in each practice site as physicians and staff care for patients. The leadership team for the organization needs to develop and approve policies and procedures to guide the operations of each practice site. The on-site leadership and management team is best able to resolve issues that involve interactions of physicians, staff, and patients in these sites. Teaming a lead physician with a lead administrator (a site manager, or a lead staff person in a smaller site) at each practice site is the way to efficiently and effectively manage daily physician, staff, and patient issues.

Political Process

Leadership and management of a medical group is a "political" process in the best sense of the word. It is the process of meeting the needs and interests of individuals in ways that also meet the collective needs and interests of the group.

The first requirement is to understand the needs and interests of each member of the group. Individuals who are new to a leadership position in medical groups will find it helpful to meet separately with each physician. The individual meetings do not need to be more than 30 to 45 minutes, but the process of meeting with each physician provides at least three positive benefits:

- The leader and each physician get to know each other on a personal basis.
- Information can be gathered on what has been working well and what needs to work better, as seen by each physician.
- Individual physicians learn that the new leader values their needs and interests.

Following these meetings, action must be taken to strike a balance between meeting the needs and interests of the individuals and those of the organization. This undertaking is not as difficult as might be imagined. However, it does mean being responsive in meeting the needs of both physicians and the organization where it is reasonably possible to do so. It also means taking time to involve physicians in issues affecting them.

Physician Involvement

Involving individual physicians in the consideration of issues affecting them has positive outcomes, as illustrated in Box 2.1.

The process of involvement takes time and the investment of leadership energy, what has been described as leadership "paying its dues." In terms of working with and involving physicians, the question is when—not if—leadership chooses to pay its dues.

It is better to have a process that engages individual physicians in wrestling with issues on the front end (Delbecq and Gill 1985). Such a process builds physician support for the decision ultimately made. Even if they disagree, physicians will understand why the decision was made.

Dr. Henry Berman (1991, p. 53), who at the time was president and CEO of Group Health Northwest, described this approach to leadership well when he described it as the authoritative style:

> The authoritative style is not a compromise between the other two styles [autocratic and laissez-faire] but a third, entirely different approach. Authoritative parents and leaders understand that they have knowledge and skills that are greater in certain areas, and responsibilities that they cannot shrug off. They also understand that wise leaders make most decisions after considerable consultation with those whom the decisions affect, that they hold as few decisions to themselves as possible, and that they encourage independent decision making.

BOX 2.1

In their article, "It Takes More Than Money," Mittyng and Wenzel (1999) discuss Park Nicollet Clinic, a large multispecialty group in Minneapolis, Minnesota. Its clinic management committee identified the importance of physician involvement by looking back and analyzing six decisions that had been made. In three cases the implementation had gone well, and in three the implementation had gone poorly. The question was: "What were the distinguishing characteristics between the implementations that went well and those that did not?" In the "good" cases the process for decision making was clearly identified at the beginning, participation was widespread and open, and the information obtained was fed back to the group so the participants would know their views had been heard and taken into account in making the decision. The decisions were supported by the group. The other three cases provided a marked contrast. The process for making the decision in these cases was not clearly identified, and information was not obtained from those affected. These decisions were not supported by the staff, and there was continuing discussion, resistance, resentment, and sabotage by those affected.

As mentioned, the leadership and management of a group of physicians is a political process. Regardless of the constituency size, leadership can get to know many people and involve most in the issues affecting them.

Mutual Agreement

If physicians see themselves as captain of the ship, the group is a ship carrying the careers of all who work there. The performance of one affects everyone else—operationally and financially. "What can I expect of you?" is a reasonable question requiring a reasonable answer from an individual interested in becoming a part of the group. A complete understanding of the answers to two questions—(1) What can you expect from me (as a leader of the group)? and (2) What can I expect from you (as a member of the group)?—is essential for success.

In a small group the individual physicians know their colleagues and their performance. Performance expectations may be written down, but often they are no more than general, unwritten understandings. In a larger group individuals may not know all of the physicians, and they know less about how well or poorly others are performing. When physicians see the group's performance affecting their future, explicit performance expectations—and incentives—become an important component of the culture (Mitlyng and Wenzel 1999).

Leadership Roles

The three top leadership positions in a medical group are the physician leader, often with the title of president; administrative leader, the person responsible for leading and managing the operations of the group; and medical director, who is responsible for overseeing the clinical care provided by the group. In the smallest groups the physician leader carries the responsibilities of all three positions with the help of an office supervisor and outside resources such as an accountant and lawyer. The largest groups have all three positions, each with support staff, and the skills of accountants and lawyers are provided by in-house staff.

Medical groups typically see the need for three separate positions when they reach a size of 50 or more physicians. The following descriptions assume three separate positions, although, as noted, in smaller groups the president may be effectively responsible for all three.

President

The president, the physician leader of the group, may have that position because he/she founded the group or has the major ownership stake in it. In most cases the president is in that position because he/she has been selected by the members of the group. The power of an elected president comes from the political legitimacy of having been chosen for the position by colleagues.

Responsibilities of the President The president is the final decision maker on all issues that do not require a decision by an executive committee or members of the group as a whole. A decision to sell the group, for example, may require a vote and approval by the members of the group. To be an effective leader of the group the president must recognize and appreciate the values of the members of the group. Responsibilities of the president include:

- lead the group in ways consistent with his/her values and the values of the group;
- lead meetings of the entire group and, in larger groups, lead the executive committee also elected by the group;
- hire the top administrative and medical leadership in the group;
- provide administrative and medical leadership for the group beyond what the other staff can provide;
- develop a strategic vision for the group that is shared by its individual members;
- develop and carry out strategic initiatives that are supported by the members of the group; and
- represent the group in dealing with the community, hospitals, and other physician groups.

Criteria for an Effective President
- Excellent clinical skills—a physician members of the group would choose to care for their family or themselves
- Values consistent with the values of most members of the group
- Good strategic and business judgment—a physician seen by his colleagues as someone who will make good decisions benefiting the group
- Articulate—someone able to communicate his vision for the future of the group and someone its members choose to follow
- Able to make the shift from clinical practice, with complete responsibility for his patients, to a shared responsibility with other leaders in the group for the success of the organization
- Willingness to take the position and do the work required to be successful in it

Administrator

The administrator is a member of the leadership team and the highest ranking business management position in the organization. The position requires someone whose expertise is in the business side of organizations and is typically not filled by a physician. The top administrative role has many titles depending on the size and form of the organization: practice manager, administrator, executive director, executive vice president, and chief operating officer.

The administrator is selected by the president and may be confirmed by vote of the executive committee in larger groups.

Responsibilities of the administrator include:

Responsibilities of the Administrator

- lead and manage the operations of the group, including its business affairs and the clinical support staff who work directly with the physicians;
- ensure that the group is profitable at year end;
- manage the business affairs and clinical support staff in a cost-effective way;
- provide support services and information meeting the needs and interests of physicians;
- take actions in her own areas of responsibility where appropriate, and recommend actions that may require the support of others where necessary to ensure a profitable year-end performance;
- lead and manage the business affairs of the group, including accounting, billing and collections, computers and information systems, facilities, human resources, and purchasing, both in relation to these support services areas as well as the clinical operations of the group;
- lead and manage, with the medical director, the workflow processes applicable to both physicians and staff;
- develop and carry out strategic initiatives in areas supported by the members of the group;
- negotiate profitable payer contracts; and
- represent the group in dealing with the community, hospitals, other physician groups, and payers.

Criteria for an Effective Administrator

- Excellent business skills—the ability to see opportunity and build value and practice profitability in the decisions she makes or recommends
- Appreciation for the values and interests of individual physicians, the group, and individual staff members
- General knowledge of all aspects of the business affairs of the group, including accounting, billing and collections, contract negotiation, human resources, and information systems, and the ability to work with experts in these areas
- Articulate—able to communicate well both in writing and in talking with individuals and groups
- Good strategic vision—able to support the physician leader in developing a strategic vision for the group
- Reasonably comfortable in dealing with ambiguity and the lack of clear direction
- Able to decide on a course of action, build support in the group as necessary, modify the course as needed to make it effective, and execute the plan to make it happen

- Strong personal values—respected by physicians, staff, and all they deal with (including hospitals, community, and payers) as both firm and fair

Clinical Medical Director

The medical director is the clinical leader of the physicians. All physicians are responsible to the medical director for the quality of care they provide, the service they provide to patients, and their relationships with colleagues and staff. The medical director is selected by the president and confirmed by the executive committee or vote of the full group.

Responsibilities of the Medical Director

Responsibilities of the medical director include:

- develop and lead the quality assurance program;
- oversee patient satisfaction surveying and provide individual performance feedback to physicians;
- lead the development and implementation of clinical information systems;
- lead and manage, with the administrator, the workflow processes applicable to both physicians and staff;
- lead the physician recruitment process;
- lead the physician compensation process (may be involved in individual physician compensation decisions); and
- deal with physician performance issues and, where necessary, lead the physician termination process.

Criteria for an Effective Medical Director

- Respected by the other physicians in the group as an excellent physician
- Recognizes and appreciates the values of members of the group
- Strong personal values—respected as firm and fair in his dealings with others
- Interest and skills in continuous quality improvement in medical care
- Experience and skills in physician recruitment, performance evaluation, and performance feedback
- Experience and skills in developing and leading a physician compensation process
- Experience and interest in the application of computer information systems to medical care
- Comfortable in dealing with physician performance issues, coaching, and termination where necessary

The responsibilities of these three positions, depending on the size of the medical group, may be held by a single physician leader, physician leader and administrator, or three separate positions in larger groups. The following section describes three common management models and the way these responsibilities are carried out in each model.

Management Models

Three management models predominate in medical groups: physician leader only, physician-administrator team, and administrator only. The following sections describe each of these models, their origins, and where they are appropriate. The choice of model depends on the interests of the physician leader, size of the group, and ownership of the group.

Physician Leader Only

Many independent medical groups start with the physician-leader-only model. Most medical groups are small, with fewer than ten physicians, and the initial business and clinical leadership is provided by the physician(s) who led the founding of the group. Some notable exceptions exist, but generally the physician-leader-only model starts with an office supervisor who oversees the office staff and billing. The business and clinical decisions in the group are all made by the physician leader.

In the smallest groups (two to five physicians) business and clinical leadership is provided by the owner or founder of the group or a member of the group who agrees to be a leader among peers. Some of the smallest groups choose to split the duties among the physicians, but the difficulties of coordinating decisions by multiple physicians rapidly make this approach unwieldy as the group grows. The key characteristic of this model is decision making only by the physician leader.

The physician leader:

- serves as both the clinical and business leader of the group;
- hires and supervises the office manager, who manages day-to-day practice operations, including support staff coverage and practice operations such as patient scheduling, rooming, support services, and billing and collections (in the smallest groups the office manager may be a working supervisor);
- provides backup support for the office manager as necessary;
- handles physician-related issues, including productivity and compensation;
- leads the group in identifying its strategic options and developing group support for those options;
- retains outside resources, including accounting and legal expertise, to meet the needs of the practice; and
- represents the group in outside relationships with the hospital and community.

In this model all members of the leadership team are physicians. All decisions are made directly (or subject to review and final decision) by the physician leader.

Physician-administrator Team

As groups grow larger, in the range of 10 to 50 physicians, the demands placed on the physician leader become more than most physicians choose to carry. The physician leader in a group of this size is expected to maintain a significant clinical practice (the *sine qua non* of "one of us") as well as see to the business affairs of the medical group. The total number of employees in a group of 10 to 50 physicians is easily 200 or more, and the business affairs become a significant challenge. The group is large enough to see the value in, and can afford, the addition of a trained and experienced full-time administrator to work as a team with the physician leader.

Leadership competence in a medical group is seen in physician leadership, particularly in relation to the clinical and political leadership needs of the group. But it is seen also in how well the business affairs of the group are managed, areas in which most physicians feel they are not competent. These areas include billing and collections, accounting and finance, computer systems, employee management, and contract negotiation. Many successful groups have found these two competencies in a physician-administrator team, which pairs the physician leader's acknowledged clinical and leadership skills with the demonstrated competence of the administrator in these other areas. The oldest, largest, best known, and most successful medical groups in the country have found the physician-administrator team model to be durable and effective.

As groups grow larger than 50 physicians, the combined clinical and political leadership role also becomes a challenge for the physician leader. The medical director position is added to the leadership team to take on some of the clinical leadership responsibilities of the physician leader. The physician leader retains responsibility for the political leadership of the group, those responsibilities that have been uniquely given to the physician leader by the members of the group. The administrator and medical director are expected to be politically astute and resolve issues in ways that minimize the need for involvement of the physician leader (now known typically as the president, with possibly the CEO title as well), but the physician leader is responsible for political issues. The physician leader cannot delegate these responsibilities and be seen as an effective leader.

For the physician-administrator team to be effective it needs to develop ways to promote frequent and open communication. In a smaller group this may be as simple as scheduling a formal meeting once a month but communicating with e-mails and by phone daily and meeting as necessary. Larger groups find it helpful to schedule weekly (or even twice weekly) meetings that include the president, administrator, medical director, vice president, and an associate administrator. In a larger group these meetings prove invaluable in ensuring the leadership team is in agreement and able to deal with issues in a coordinated and timely way.

Administrator Leader Only

Physicians value physician leadership. Physician leaders are seen as people who are (or at least at one time were) "one of us." Some hospital-owned groups have tried to put an administrator in the lead position. Hospitals have used this model in other relationships with physicians (e.g., hospital product line managers), and trying this approach has been a logical step for hospital leadership.

Taking sole responsibility for leadership of a medical group is a tough challenge. The sole leader is seen as responsible for every problem that occurs in the group (Berman 1991), a particularly difficult challenge for an administrator. The administrator cannot satisfy the fundamental interest of physicians in having a physician leader. An administrator in that position is well-advised to develop a relationship with a physician leader/medical director to form a physician-administrator team.

Keys to Success

Three elements are required for a successful physician group:

1. understanding the interests and values of physicians who are members of the group;
2. a competent leadership team; and
3. the ability of the group to support the practice of the individual physicians in ways they value.

The following sections address each of these elements.

Understanding Physician Interests and Values

Physicians are commonly viewed as bright, highly educated, and highly motivated people. They are also often viewed as highly motivated by money, but the reality is a far more complex set of interests and values (Mitlyng and Wenzel 1999), which for most physicians include:

- providing the best care for their patients;
- personal control over what they do and how they practice;
- limited control by others;
- doing well in comparison with peers;
- sense of fairness in relationships;
- environment of clinical inquiry;
- opportunity for dialogue;
- collegial relations with peers;
- choice of those with whom they work; and
- partnership model.

Creating a Competent Leadership Team

The basic capabilities required to lead a medical group are outlined above in the descriptions of the three leadership positions. Leadership demonstrates competence to the medical group members in how well the group does on the basics—managing the clinical and business affairs well. High-quality care must be a top priority, and continued bottom-line profitability will carry the leadership team a long way.

But what happens when continued bottom-line profitability depends on changes affecting how each physician practices? Just proposing those changes is a threat to the highest physician values. Accomplishing them requires engaging each physician in making the necessary changes in how they practice. In large part, leadership competence today is demonstrated by how well the leadership and management team works with physicians, engaging each physician in making the changes required for the group to succeed.

Support for Individual Physicians

Most physicians share the core set of values outlined above. In addition to having those values met, individuals also need to feel they are receiving reasonable compensation for their work.

What is seen as reasonable compensation by individual physicians ranges widely depending on their interests. Depending on the individual, reasonable compensation can take many forms:

- compensation the individual considers competitive with what they can earn elsewhere;
- appropriate amounts of personal time to spend as they choose;
- good daily practice environment (competence of the staff and quality of the group's facilities, equipment, and systems); or
- opportunities to teach or do research.

Some groups focus on maximizing dollar compensation, whereas others focus on what they see as lifestyle. Still others choose to make major investments in the development of the group to add more services for patients, add facilities and equipment, and improve the competence and efficiency of the services supporting their practice; other groups have a significant commitment to teaching and research. It is important to recruit new members who share the group's values.

Identifying the appropriate compensation for individuals in the group requires the leadership team to recognize and appreciate the predominant compensation values of physicians in the group. Dealing with the interests of individual physicians, in ways consistent with the values of the group, is an ongoing challenge for physician group leadership.

Effective Decision-making Process

This section summarizes the two essential elements of an effective decision-making process in a physician group. Who makes the decision and how the decision is made are critical to effective decision making. As in Box 2.1, an effective decision is one that was supported by the group and accomplished what was intended. Appendix 2.1 presents a series of effective and ineffective ways of handling some common issues.

Who Makes the Decision?

Earlier in this chapter an effective decision-making process is described as a political process in the best sense. The corollary is that effective decisions are made by those seen as having the expertise to make them. The administrator and administrative staff are seen as having expertise in the business affairs of the group—billing and collections, accounting and finance, computer systems, employee management, contract negotiation, and marketing. The administrator, as part of the physician-administrator team, is expected to take the lead in those areas and, depending on the potential impact of the decision, be sure the physician leader is aware of the choices and the rationale behind them.

How Is the Decision Made?

In even the business affairs areas it is important that other members of the leadership team experience no surprises. In all other areas making effective decisions requires involving representatives of groups that will be affected by the decision. Physicians need to be involved when the decision will affect physicians.

Summary

The leadership and management of a physician group is a political process. Effective leaders and managers know the needs and interests of individuals as well as the needs and interests of the group. They involve individuals in decisions affecting them and make final decisions in ways that reasonably meet the needs and interests of both the group and its individual members.

Discussion Questions

1. How does the concept of captain of the ship influence leading and managing physician groups?
2. Describe the roles of the three principal leadership positions and their effect on the success of the physician organization.

3. How do the politics of the group affect the leadership and management of the organization?
4. What criteria are most important in deciding the who and how of decisions that will be made in the group? What influence will these criteria have on the process?

References

Berman, H. 1991. "Commentary: Reflections of a Seasoned Veteran." In *My Pulse Is Not what it Used to Be*, edited by C. R. Fernandez and I. M. Rubin, 52–58. Honolulu: The Temenos Foundation..

Delbecq, A. L., and S. L. Gill. 1985. "Justice as a Prelude to Teamwork in Medical Centers." *Health Care Management Review* 10 (1): 45–51.

Mitlyng, J. W., and F. J. Wenzel. 1999. "It Takes More than Money—Keys to Success in Leading and Managing Physician Groups." *Medical Group Management Journal* 46 (2): A30–38.

Medical Group Management Association. 2003. "Performances and Practices of Successful Medical Groups." 2002 report based on 2001 data. Denver: Medical Group Management Association.

APPENDIX 2.1. EXAMPLES OF COMMON ISSUES AND DECISION-MAKING PROCESSES

Developing a Budget

Ineffective process	*Effective process*
The administrator and finance staff develop the budget without involving the physicians and present the budget to the governing board for approval. Individual physicians, specialty areas, and offices see it as "administration's budget"; there is no ownership of budget performance outside of administration.	The administrator and finance staff meet with the physician leader and supporting manager in each specialty or office in the organization to review draft budgets prepared by the physician leader and her supporting manager. Local specialty area or office ownership for budget performance is developed as part of the process.

"Accounting" for the group's performance is a purely administrative responsibility. Developing a budget that includes expectations for physician productivity and how the group's dollars will be spent requires involvement by physicians.

Improving Physician Productivity

Ineffective process	*Effective process*
The president and the administrator meet with the members of the group and say the group is losing money. If the physicians add just one more patient per day, the group will be profitable. No explanation of the possible impact of factors other than individual physician productivity is given; revenue factors such as decline in reimbursement rates, business office collection performance, or number of patients available to be seen; or possible increases in expenses such as staffing, malpractice insurance, or overhead are not discussed.	The president and administrator meet with the group and say the group's financial performance is dropping, before the group is actually losing money if possible; it helps to have time to change. The president and administrator present their analysis of the possible factors other than physician productivity contributing to the loss. The physicians are asked to contribute their thinking on changes to improve financial performance, and the administrative staff analyzes any added possible changes that have not already been considered.

When increasing physician productivity or decreasing physician compensation are the only significant variables left, each physician will choose what will meet the needs of the group and work best for them.

Changing the Physician Compensation System

Ineffective process

The president and administrator develop a new compensation plan and present it to the group as "the new compensation plan." This approach can work if the president is the sole owner of the group and the physicians in the group are satisfied with their compensation.

Effective process

The president reviews the problems with the present compensation plan with the group, then appoints a panel of respected members to work with the president and administrator as the compensation plan committee. The plan developed with the committee, and the reasoning behind the choices made, is presented to the group for approval.

A senior physician in a large physician group once said, "There is no such thing as an equitable compensation plan. The best you can hope for is an acceptable plan."

Managing Staffing Costs: Numbers of Staff and Wage Levels

Less effective process

Staff managers develop justifications for the added staff or added compensation. The decisions to add staff and increase staff compensation levels are made by the administrator or other senior administrative staff. The decision process is a tug of war between the physician or manager wanting to add staff or staff compensation and the administrator.

More effective process

The physicians' compensation system is tied to the direct costs of their practices, including the cost of support staff. This gives them the option to add staff or to add staff responsibilities and compensation. Physicians in groups, as in private practice, make sound economic decisions when the benefits and costs of those decisions come back to them.

Interestingly, MGMA groups reporting better financial performance have higher than median staffing levels (MGMA, 2003). The conclusion is that these groups have more staff and make better use of their staff to improve the financial performance of the group. In either approach above, the development of a clearly articulated workflow model will aid and improve the decision making; the strength of the more effective process is in the ability of the physicians with compensation at risk to make changes they see will improve their overall performance.

Constructing a New Building or Major Addition

Less effective process

The president and the administrator announce to the group that the organization needs more space, and ABC Architects have been engaged to begin drawing up the plans.

More effective process

The president and administrator begin talking about the issues and problems with the current space. The president appoints a building committee to work with a building consultant to develop a program plan for new space. The consultant works with members of the building committee and meets with each clinical and support services area to identify the added space needs in each area. The cost for constructing the total added space identified is estimated, compared to what the group can afford, and reviewed with the group's leadership for approval. The building committee presents its recommended plan for the added space and the estimated construction cost to the group for approval.

Buying a New Computer System

Less effective process

The administrator and senior administrative staff look at the major systems available and decide which system provides the best value for the group—the best combination of benefits and price. The administrator

More effective process

The administrator identifies the types of positions whose work will be affected by the new computer system and appoints a computer selection committee with membership representing the various positions.

presents the recommendation to the president (and the group if required) for approval.

The individuals appointed are chosen because they are respected by their colleagues. Key physicians are also asked to serve on the committee, which is chaired by a senior administrator and reports to the administrator. The recommendation resulting from the committee's work is presented to the president and the group for approval.

Buying a New CT Scanner

Less effective process

The radiologists or other physicians interested in the group's purchase of a new CT scanner look at the choices and present their recommendation to the group for approval.

More effective process

The radiologists or other physicians interested in the group's purchase of a new CT scanner look at the choices and present them, with supporting analysis and rationale, to the administrator. The administrator assists the interested physicians in evaluating the choices and developing a recommendation to present to the group.

Measuring Clinical Care Quality and Taking Corrective Action as Necessary

Less effective process

Hire staff to perform the process of measuring quality and identify an interested physician to work with this staff. Have this staff report to the medical director, but leave it to the staff to meet with individual physicians and provide feedback on an advisory basis.

More effective process

Do the same, but tie physician compensation to meeting minimum performance expectations.

Deciding Which Billing Clerk to Hire

Less effective process	*More effective process*
Have someone not responsible for the billing area, possibly someone in human resources, interview the candidates and decide which one to hire.	Have human resources screen the candidates for minimum qualifications, but send the candidates to the manager of billing to decide which candidate to hire.

Deciding Which Medical Assistant to Hire

Less effective process	*More effective process*
Have human resources screen the candidates, but then send the candidates to the administrative person to whom the medical assistant will report for a decision on who to hire.	Do the same, but have the physician with whom the medical assistant will be working interview the final candidates. Even a brief meeting between the physician and medical assistant gives each a chance to decide in advance if they are likely to work well together.

Deciding Which Physician to Hire

Less effective process	*More effective process*
The president, medical director, and administrator interview the candidates and decide who to hire. The candidates may visit with physicians in the group to talk about the practice, but the president decides both whom to hire and where they will practice in the group.	The president, medical director, and administrator interview the candidates and decide which candidates to send on to meet with the physicians in the group who want to recruit a new partner for the practice. Openings for new physicians are seen in the context of openings with the physicians in a particular office or specialty. No offer is made to a candidate unless the physicians with at least one of the openings say they want that

candidate to join their practice. The result is physician practices staffed with physicians who see each other as colleagues and who have chosen to work together.

Deciding to Terminate an Employee

Less effective process

Notice that the employee is not performing up to expectations, but do not document the performance or take corrective action. Eventually a specific event necessitates immediate termination. The needed documentation is not there, and the individual who should have been fired outright instead leaves with a severance package.

More effective process

Make documentation of employee performance—both good and bad—a leadership and management priority. Insisting an employee be fired without adequate evidence of due process should be a reason to discipline the employee's manager.

Deciding to Terminate a Physician

Less effective process

Notice the physician is not living up to expectations, but do not document performance or take corrective action. Also do not raise the issue of a performance problem (on a need-to-know and confidential basis) with other members of the leadership team or physician leaders in the group. Eventually a specific event necessitates immediate termination. Not only is the needed documentation not there, but the members of the group who have no knowledge of the situation rally to the support of their colleague who is (apparently) being treated unjustly. A contest between the individual and the

More effective process

Make documentation of physician performance—both good and bad—a leadership and management priority, and make a corrective action plan in any instances of documented poor performance. The financial stakes of a six-month or one-year severance are too high to not have the leadership team accountable to one another and to the group for effective, timely action in dealing with poor performance. This is also the fairest way to deal with the individual involved.

leader of the group can develop. Getting rid of the individual may be much more difficult, time consuming, and expensive than necessary.

Identifying Opportunities to Add Clinical Services

Less effective process

Add a service that someone in the group, possibly an influential physician, decides would be worthwhile. Do no analysis of the market for the service, including the competitors and their likely response to the new service, likely revenues, or likely expenses and operating contribution of the new service.

More effective process

Do the market and financial analysis outlined. It may serve only to confirm a conclusion to add the service, but doing the analysis will likely raise questions. The process of answering the questions will provide insights as to steps that can be taken to increase the likelihood of the project's success.

Identifying Opportunities to Add Offices

Less effective process

Decide to locate offices because if the group does not, someone else will.

More effective process

Do the analysis. Identify opportunities to retain or grow market share, set performance expectations, measure actual performance, and review performance at least annually. Take corrective action where indicated.

Measuring Patient Satisfaction, Providing Feedback, and Taking Corrective Action

Less effective process

Hire staff to perform the process of measuring patient satisfaction and identify an interested physician to work with this staff. Have this staff report to the medical director,

More effective process

Do the same, but tie physician compensation to meeting minimum performance expectations.

but leave it to the staff to meet with individual physicians and provide feedback on an advisory basis.

Measuring Staff Satisfaction, Providing Feedback, and Taking Corrective Action

Less effective process	*More effective process*
Make this measurement, feedback, and corrective action process the responsibility of human resources.	Use the results of measuring staff satisfaction as the basis for at least annual meetings between the administrator and groups of employees. Having these meetings, and using them for the administrator to talk about the issues and the constructive steps being taken, provides the basis for a strong culture in which the administrator (and the organization) values each employee.

Measuring Physician Satisfaction, Providing Feedback, and Taking Corrective Action

Less effective process	*More effective process*
Assume everyone who has not left the organization is satisfied with the organization. Do not survey the physicians.	Survey physician satisfaction at least annually. Use the results for meetings by the president and administrator with each group of physicians to talk about the issues and corrective actions being taken. As with staff, these meetings provide the basis for a strong culture that values each physician.

Reviewing Physician Performance

Less effective process	*More effective process*
Do not perform physician performance review. Focus only on performance issues as they arise.	Perform physician performance review at least annually using a "360-degree" process with input

from the leader to whom the physician reports, other physicians and professional staff with whom the physician works, and staff who work for the physician. The president or medical director meets with each physician and discusses the physician's plan to improve performance.

Reviewing Physician Performance

Less effective process

Have the manager keep notes on things the employee is doing well and things they could improve. Summarize the notes and review them with the employee as part of their annual review.

More effective process

The manager for each staff member should review the information on what is working and what could be working better with the staff member as the information is known. Use the 360-degree process at least annually to give employees feedback on how their performance is viewed by those to whom they report, those with whom they work, and (for managers) those who report to them.

GOVERNANCE ORGANIZATIONAL MODELS AND ISSUES

Frederick J. Wenzel

Learning Objectives

This chapter will enable the reader to:

- understand the structural perspectives of the organization based on its professional and management functions;
- place in perspective those legal and regulatory issues unique to group practices;
- understand the role organizational culture plays in determining the ability of the group to not only protect itself, but also to implement change process; and
- understand the origins and definition of conflict and ways in which the resolution process can be implemented.

Chapter Purpose

One of the key factors that will promote the understanding of group practice is an appreciation of the unique characteristics of the professional organization. The structure, organization, and function of these organizations are such that the standards of the profession frequently conflict with the complexity of the organization and its needs. Historically, professional autonomy extended to the expectation that there would be complete freedom to conduct the business affairs of the organization and each individual could make his own decision about how the group should function. That uniqueness remains, but shifts in recent years have been brought on by the need for professionals to be financially and legally accountable for the performance of their organizations. This chapter describes the organizational models groups have adopted to serve as the core of their operations and issues related to culture, structure, and legal implications in detail. Professional liability is considered, with emphasis on medical practice restrictions and constraints that result from legislation and regulation. Conflict is also covered, especially as it relates to the ever-changing medical care environment. Conflict between the professionals and the organization, especially the management staff, is described, and resolution measures are proposed.

Case in Point

Jim Dunn is the CEO of the Merryville multispecialty clinic. One busy Monday morning his assistant entered his office with a worried look on her face. "There is a lawyer here to see you about a patient of one of our doctors. Should I tell him you are out?" Jim frowned and said, "No, tell him that I will see him in a few minutes." The assistant left the office and appeared five minutes later, introducing Paul Hughes, attorney at law. The lawyer told Jim that he had a request for information (the medical record) signed by one of the clinic's patients, and he wished to have a copy of the patient's medical record. Just then the lawyer's cell phone rang. He answered and asked Jim if he could take a few minutes to answer an important call. Jim said that would be fine, giving himself a few minutes to think about how to handle the request. He pondered his next move as the lawyer stepped into the adjoining room. Should he call Merryville's attorney for advice? Should he simply provide Mr. Hughes with the information he wanted? Should he call the patient and verify the request? What do you think the appropriate response would be?

Organization Models—Structure

As most readers will already have been exposed to healthcare law in a broad sense, this section deals principally with those organizations and corporations in which physician groups are housed. These take a number of forms or structures, including sole proprietor or solo practice, partnerships, corporations, limited liability corporations, and foundations. The type of structure will often be determined by the size and mission of the physician organization. Understanding the corporate structure of the physician organization is important because the law and regulations as they apply to these organizations are different, and an understanding of the relationship of these laws and regulations is an important aspect of the manager's responsibilities.

Sole Proprietorships

The sole proprietor is the simplest model for a medical service organization. It is not a true organization in the usual sense, but for tax purposes it bears the name sole proprietorship. The physician owns the practice, which is a for-profit entity, and she bears full responsibility for the delivery of care as well as the legal and financial issues related to the practice. The physician makes all the decisions related to the practice and its development, and as long as all of the practice actions are within the law and the practice is financially viable the individual enjoys a great deal of freedom. This form of medical practice was at one time common, but it has become rare as the delivery of medical services becomes more complex.

Partnerships

Partnerships are governed by state law and the agreements that have been prepared between the individuals in the partnership. These agreements have great latitude and are constructed according to the needs of the partners and their organization. The partners agree to receive equal shares of profits or losses, are entitled to equal voting rights, and are personally liable for the debts of the venture in most partnerships. The partnership on its surface appears to be less complex than the corporation, and it is characteristically found in a number of single-specialty physician groups. While the organization may have other members, the business is controlled by the owner partners. Most partnerships are organized under subchapter S of the statutes and are frequently called S organizations. These partnerships have a significant advantage over the corporation because the partners are taxed individually. In contrast the corporation is taxed and then, should there be a dividend or distribution of profits, individuals are taxed again. This is referred to as double taxation (Harris 2003). Liability, however, is shared equally among the partners.

There are also limited partnerships in which the general partner has responsibility for liabilities of the partnership. The general partner also has control.

Corporations, Professional Corporations, Professional Associations, and Service Corporations

Most group practices, especially larger groups and multispecialty organizations, form for-profit corporations that in many cases are called professional corporations (PC), professional associations (PA), or service corporations (SC). These organizations bear responsibility for legal issues and debts and pay corporate taxes at the federal and state level as well. The advantage of the corporation is the limitation on the liability of the individual physician; however, double taxation is a disadvantage.

Physician corporations ordinarily move physicians to shareholder status after a set period as an associate, during which time the physician is under contract. The shareholders elect a board of directors from their number that is responsible for the governance of the organization according to the powers delegated to it by the shareholders. In large boards, an executive committee may be responsible for the day-to-day operation of the organization. Typically in small physician groups all shareholders are on the board of directors, which can make governance of the organization unwieldy. Often the share-

FIGURE 3.1

Relationship Between Personal Liability and Tax Advantage

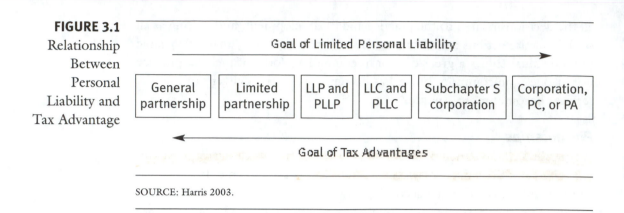

SOURCE: Harris 2003.

holders are unwilling to give up their involvement in policymaking, which leads to a lack of consensus and a slow-moving organization. Another issue related to the corporation model is that directors may become involved in the management of the organization, leading to confusion and managerial problems. More than one manager has lost his position because of confrontations with the board on management rather than policy issues.

Limited Liability Companies

The limited liability company (LLC) is a relatively new hybrid organization that may be used for joint ventures. Each participating organization has an ownership interest, and this model is a way to develop partnerships between a physician organization and a hospital. The for-profit corporation contributes certain assets to the jointly owned LLC, and the not-for-profit organization may contribute its operating assets. The LLC is like a corporation in terms of its liability, but it is taxed like a partnership. It has more flexibility than a subchapter S corporation.

Figure 3.1 shows the reciprocal relationship of the limited personal liability and tax advantage goals. Personal liability of the individual in a corporation is less than in a partnership. The tax advantage to the individual is less in the corporation and greater in the partnership.

Foundations

Foundations are not-for-profit organizations qualified under 501(c)(3) of the federal tax code. These organizations, called charitable trusts, must devote a substantial part of their mission to research and education and other public good in order to be qualified. Hospitals are typically recognized as not-for-profits under this section of the statute. More and more large multispecialty clinics are also being qualified under this section of the code. Along with the advantage of not-for-profit status, which means foundations do not pay corporate tax, is the opportunity to accept charitable contributions and participate in tax-exempt financing. There also exists a provision that there shall be no inurement to the members of the organization for being part of the delivery system. 1996 revisions in the tax code call for an excise tax to be levied against those corporations and individuals who profit from being members of the organization or had compensation levels outside market-place levels. Thus far, few cases have reached the courts.

Faculty practice plans, the organizational component and legal structure of the departments of medical schools, are qualified under 501(c)(3), making them not-for-profit. More recently, however, more medical schools are forming foundations to deal with the complexity of the healthcare system, especially compliance and reimbursement.

Professional Organizations

Fogel (1989) describes a number of unique characteristics of the professional organization. He defines the organization as a professional bureaucracy with the characteristics shown in Figure 3.2 (1989, p. 16).

Fogel (1989, p. 20) further emphasizes 12 points for managing physicians effectively (see Figure 3.3). Managers who understand these principles will be successful managing and will meet the needs of the patients, physicians, and organization. Those who do not understand the principles will find management difficult and eventually leave the practice. This task is much easier in organizations led by a physician-manager team, in which a common understanding of the professional bureaucracy is much easier to reach. The efficient functioning of this team is described in Chapter 2.

Legal Issues

The legal issues cited in this chapter are limited to those that affect group practices. While the principal legal issues seem to be professional liability and antitrust, there exist a number of other legal questions, collectively called the Corporate Compliance Acts (CCA), related to fraud and abuse, false claims, kickbacks, the Stark self-referral laws, and the Health Insurance Portability and Accountability Act (HIPAA). Because the government is the

---

- Standard set of skills shared by the professionals.
- Organization is decentralized.
- Marketing and functional units operate side by side.
- Bureaucracy serves the professionals and relies on their skills and knowledge.
- Organization produces standardized products and services.
- Keys to success are service and expertise.

FIGURE 3.2
Unique Characteristics of the Professional Bureaucracy

FIGURE 3.3

What Managers
Need to
Know About
Physicians

1. Physicians are trained to operate independently.

2. Power rests with the physicians.

3. Physicians join organizations for shared resources and skill enhancement.

4. Work is coordinated and enhanced primarily through standard routines, communication, and knowledge shared among professionals.

5. Control is extremely difficult.

6. Patient has certain powers of coordination.

7. Bureaucracy is set up to serve the physicians' needs.

8. Key executives are powerful only when they are perceived to be serving the physicians.

9. Marketing is the province of each professional as well as the organization.

10. Innovation and change are difficult to achieve.

11. Successful professional bureaucracies give preference to professional goals over bureaucratic rules.

12. Selection of physicians is the most important organizational process.

largest single purchaser of healthcare, Medicare has been the origin of most of this legislation and regulation since the early 1970s.

Professional Liability

The physician-patient relationship may be established by an expressed or implied contract. An implied contract exists when a physician agrees to see a patient by making an appointment. Professional liability arises when the patient believes the contract has been breached; the physician did not adhere to his agreement in the implied contract for care. While most professional liability cases arise because of alleged negligence, malpractice suits can include intentional torts or breach of contract (Showalter 2003). A tort is an intentional wrong that results in an injury (it is not necessarily a breach of contract). There are far fewer actions related to intentional torts than to negligence. Negligence may arise from either omission or commission. Figure 3.4 shows some of the key reasons for malpractice actions.

Negligence is generally the most common cause for action in a professional liability case. Showalter (2003) stated that four elements are essential to prove negligence: duty of due care, breach of duty, causation, and damages. These elements relate to a number of different standards of care that may be based on community, state, or federal standards. The standard of care is defined as follows: "A physician is bound to bestow such reasonable and ordinary care, skill, and diligence as physicians and surgeons in good standing in the same neighborhood, in the same general line of practice, ordinarily have and exercise in similar cases" (Showalter 2003, p. 39). The local or community standard appears in virtually all cases in which there is an allegation of negligence.

Premiums for professional liability insurance have risen sharply over the last 25 years, and it is not unusual for a physician to leave her home state to practice in another state where the malpractice premiums are lower. Some communities have lost obstetrical and gynecological services because of the professional liability premiums for these services; the same is true for many surgical specialties as well as anesthesia. Some states are legislating maximums that place caps on malpractice awards, especially noneconomic claims.

It is incumbent on the manager to have a full understanding of the ramifications of professional liability and malpractice potential. All organizations should have a well-established incident-reporting system, which should be evaluated on a periodic basis. Anything out of the ordinary should be reported by all staff members on a standard form, with assurance that the reporting person will be protected. These reports are reviewed by the medical director and legal counsel. This will eliminate surprises, and should a certain type of incident increase, preventive measures can be taken to deal with the situation. Incident reporting is an important management tool and can, if done properly, materially reduce the potential for professional liability claims.

FIGURE 3.4
Key Reasons for Professional Liability Actions

Duty arising from the physician-patient relationship: the patient had an alleged adverse outcome or the physician did not order a test or procedure

Termination of the relationship: the physician discharged the patient from her care

Breach of contract: failure to perform a service with reasonable skill

Breach of warranty: physician makes a promise that was not kept

Intentional tort: a civil wrong not based on contract that results in injury

Assault and battery: concern about being touched in an insulting way, provoking physical injury

Defamation: injury to a person's reputation

False imprisonment: holding a person against his will

Invasion of privacy or wrongful disclosure of confidential information: subjecting the patient to unwanted publicity or disclosure of private information

Misrepresentation: a fact was falsely presented

Outrage: extreme or outrageous conduct

Violation of civil rights: failure to treat a patient because of race or ethnicity

The manager must also be aware of his responsibilities when a lawyer appears in the office asking for a patient's records. The manager is responsible for ensuring that the matter is placed in the hands of the appropriate personnel, usually the medical director and general counsel. A manager and medical director working together to promote an environment of good patient relationships can reduce the number of professional liability actions. Leadership and management of the organization must take a proactive position in the face of an increasingly litigious society.

Antitrust

A number of statutes are related to antitrust, including the Sherman Act passed by congress in 1890, the Clayton Act of 1914, and the Federal Trade Commission Act passed in 1914. There have also been a number of amendments; the first, to the Clayton Act, is the Robinson-Pattman Act of 1936. This act prohibits activities that result in discriminatory pricing. There have been other amendments, most recently the Celler-Kefauver Act passed in 1950.

Sherman Act Section 1 of the Sherman Act states:

> Every contract, combination in the form of trust or otherwise, or conspiracy, in restraint of trade or commerce among the several states, or with foreign nations, is hereby declared to be illegal. Every person who shall make any contract or engage in any combination or conspiracy hereby declared to be illegal shall be deemed guilty of a felony, and, upon conviction thereof, shall be punished by fines not exceeding $1 million if a corporation, or, if any other person, $100,000, or by imprisonment not exceeding three years or by both said punishments, in the discretion of the court (15 U.S.C. S 1; cited in Showalter 2003, p. 197).

Section 2 refers to a unilateral action of a single firm or business enterprise to form a monopoly, or attempts in conjunction with another organization or person to monopolize a market. It is important to note that in a case of violation of Section 2, "The court must establish the relevant geographic market for the product; determine if the evidence demonstrates real or inferred control of prices or exclusion of competitors; and determine if this monopoly power was acquired or maintained willfully" (cited in Showalter 2003, p. 199).

Clayton Act The Clayton Act came about to deal with some of the specifics of the antitrust activity, including price discrimination. When the act was amended by Robinson Pattman in 1926, it read:

> Is it is unlawful to discriminate in price between different purchasers of commodities of any like grade and quality...where the effect of such discrimination

may substantially lessen competition or tend to create a monopoly in any line of commerce, or to injure, destroy, or prevent competition with any person who either grants or knowingly receives the benefit from such discrimination (cited in Showalter 2003, p. 184).

Section 3 of the act prohibits tying and exclusive dealing. Tying is a legal or moral obligation to someone or something typically constituting a restraining power, influence, or duty. Exclusive dealing is an important consideration for group practices, as they contract with hospitals or other providers. It has been stated that healthcare organizations can be treated differently than other industries when dealing with antitrust issues. A doctrine of implied repeal suggests that if the organization has as its goals improving the health of the community; increasing the accessibility, acceptability, continuity, and quality of health services; restraining increase in the costs of health services; and preventing unnecessary duplication of health resources, there may be a case for exemption. The final word, however, is decided in the courts.

For some time it was assumed the Federal Trade Commission did not have jurisdiction over not-for-profit entities; however, in a number of cases, especially the Rockford Memorial case (15 U.S.C. S 21), the Court explained that mergers could be exempt only in regulated industries. The exemption was determined not to apply to not-for-profit organizations such as clinics or hospitals.

The lesson for managers is to be careful about mergers and acquisitions and be especially careful when contracting and providing pricing information. Consultation with legal counsel is always recommended.

Corporate Compliance

Every organization should have a corporate compliance program that includes the elements listed in Figure 3.5 (Showalter 2003, p. 231). There should be a corporate compliance committee, and one of its members should be the organization's general counsel. Smaller practices may use

---

- Compliance standards and procedures overseen at a high level within the organization.

- Policy requiring criminal background checks.

- Effective communication of standards of conduct.

- Methods to ensure how compliance will be achieved.

- In cases where discipline is necessary it should be appropriate and consistent.

- Response to violations must be appropriate and consistent.

FIGURE 3.5

Important Elements of a Corporate Compliance Program

FIGURE 3.6

Benefits of a
Corporate
Compliance
Plan

- Identify weaknesses in internal systems and management.

- Demonstrate the organization's strong commitment to honest and responsible corporate conduct.

- Provide a more accurate view of employee and contractor behavior relating to fraud and abuse.

- Identify and prevent criminal and unethical conduct.

- Improve the quality of patient care.

- Create a centralized source for distributing information and healthcare statutes and regulations.

- Develop a process that allows employees to report potential problems.

- Develop procedures that allow prompt, thorough investigation of alleged misconduct.

- Initiate immediate and appropriate corrective action.

- Minimize the loss to the government from false claims and thus reduce the organization's exposure to civil damages and penalties, criminal sanctions, and administrative remedies such as program exclusion.

outside counsel to fill that role. Figure 3.6 outlines the benefits of a well-managed corporate compliance plan (Showalter 2003).

The following areas are generally covered by the Corporate Compliance Acts:

- **False claims**, defined as knowingly presenting a false or fraudulent claim to the government for payment, or maintaining false records.
- **Kickbacks**, or payments to a provider to induce referrals.
- **Stark laws I and II**, violations that are complicated; to understand them one must use a case-by-case analysis. Briefly, they prohibit a physician or other providers from referring Medicare or Medicaid patients for certain services in which the provider or her family has a financial interest. A variety of services are covered, including:

  —clinical laboratory;
  —radiology;
  —radiation therapy;
  —physical and occupational therapy;
  —durable medical goods;
  —parenteral and enteral equipment and supplies;
  —prosthetics, orthotics, and prosthetic devices and supplies;
  —outpatient drugs;
  —home health services; and
  —inpatient and outpatient hospital services.

Violations of the Stark laws are serious and can incur denial of payment for the services, an obligation to refund, civil monetary penalties, and potentially exclusion from the Medicare and Medicaid programs.

Health Insurance Portability and Accountability Act (HIPAA)

HIPAA is the most recent of the laws passed by congress, and it has had a profound impact on group practices and other healthcare organizations. The act provides patients with more control over their health information, restricts and limits the use and disclosure of medical records, provides safeguards to protect the privacy of health information, and stipulates that violators will be held accountable through civil and criminal penalties.

Providers and health plans are obligated to notify patients of their privacy rights, and virtually all healthcare organizations have patients sign a form stating that they have been informed about their right to privacy, with significant detail about how their healthcare information may be used. Certain uses and disclosures are not restricted; these uses in general are those required by law or for legal purposes.

It is incumbent on the organization to ensure that proper policies and procedures are in place and staff are trained in the requirements imposed by law. A compliance officer should be appointed to ensure that all of the requirements are being met. The compliance officer should make periodic reports to the board of directors. Thus the new culture of confidentiality must be espoused by all healthcare organizations.

Culture and the Organization

Definition of Culture

The culture of the organization has a profound effect on all of its activities and functions, including clinical, governance, managerial, and business operations. There are a number of definitions of culture, but it can best be summed up as "the way we do things around here" (Wenzel 1989). Culture has also been characterized as a system of shared beliefs, values, and behaviors. It has a strong relationship to the norms, values, and unwritten rules of conduct of the organization. An inquiry into the culture of an organization might look at the management style, priorities, beliefs, and interpersonal behavior of everyone in the organization. There are also the stories of idols past and present that describe the institution. All of these elements are buried deep in the fabric of the organization, and they make up its culture.

The organization's culture can act as an inertial guidance system to keep it on an even keel, but it can be a double-edged sword. Culture can provide defense for the organization should it be challenged, but it can also resist needed change. It is essential that the manager have a complete under-

BOX 3.1

> A typical example is the case of a crisis in the emergency department. The doctors in the department had contracted as a group with the hospital for more than 30 years. During that time they worked with the hospital's nurses and other staff, forming strong relationships. The hospital was not entirely happy with the emergency department physician group because of its apparent lack of interest in the hospital's value systems. The hospital decided to bring in a new emergency department physician group and did so with little preparation or appreciation of the cultural implications. The hospital encountered a significant cultural barrier—the relationships between the members of the emergency department staff. The result was a significant conflict that ended with the hospital retaining the original group. The culture (the way we do things around here) was so strong that it successfully resisted the change.

standing of the organization's culture before developing any change process (see Box 3.1).

Characteristics of Culture

Virtually all organizations have a dominant culture surrounded by a variety of subcultures. Typically departments of larger hospitals and clinics have a strong measure of their own goals and ways of doing things. As long as these subcultures overlap significantly with the dominant culture the organization has a relatively stable cultural orientation. The other aspect of organizational culture is the counterculture, which generally does not overlap with the dominant culture and can provide a real challenge to leadership and management. One must be careful in dealing with the counterculture too harshly because innovation and new ideas frequently have their origins there.

Understanding Culture

There is no question that we need to understand the culture of the organization, especially if the organization is involved in a change process. Culture acts as a silent governor. When new strategies are being planned, the culture of the organization must be considered. There are a number of approaches to dealing with culture:

1. change it;
2. manage around it; or
3. develop strategic positions that fit the organization's culture.

The first and third are viable options, whereas the second is difficult and expensive.

A good understanding of an organization's culture can be gained through the answers to the following questions:

1. **What are the major events in the organization's past?** They might include the change from the president founder, a benevolent dictator, to an individual with a strong democratic bent.
2. **What does the organization stands for?** For instance, the organization states and believes "the patient comes first."
3. **How do individuals first learn about their positions within the organization?** The organization has a well-structured orientation program.
4. **What factors have high and low priorities within the organization?** For instance, the organization places high priority on the delivery of quality health services.

Changing the Culture

A corporate culture profile can be prepared by developing a perspective of the existing culture through examination of the organization's documents, systems, and strategies. Next, the desired culture can be defined by determining the ideal culture. For example, all staff members are exceedingly sensitive to the needs of the patients and work together to fulfill those needs. This tone was set by the new CEO, and she led the group by example to make it part of the fabric of the organization. Then, the present culture must be evaluated to find out what is behind the way we do things around here. The final step is to formulate recommendations for change in the culture and develop systems that will favorably position the organization and provide it with a better opportunity to achieve its long-term goals. The CEO in this example saw a good organization, focused its efforts, and slowly changed the culture to the point where everyone was the best they could be.

In order to understand culture one must also understand the potential for corporate culture failure and its impact on change. Failure is related to a number of factors, including soft commitment by the organization's leadership, adherence to traditional win-lose attitudes, inadequate involvement at all staff levels, inefficient attention to middle management, inappropriate pace or level of expectation, and failure to internalize the change process.

Leadership and Management Implications

The physician leader and manager must understand the culture of their organization if they are to be successful, especially in the strategic planning and change processes. Leaders must have a clear understanding of those things that make the organization tick, sometimes a difficult goal to achieve. We all have mental models of what we believe the organization and its principals are; while those mental models may be shared by some, they may not be shared by all. This follows from a lack of understanding of the culture of the organization and eventually leads to conflict. Leadership and management should become students of the professional organization. Through a committed study of the organization and its culture they will become knowledgeable on how both can work together toward achieving the organization's mission and vision.

Conflict

All of the issues discussed in this chapter are sure to promote the development of conflict within the organization. It is therefore important that the manager develop a process for conflict resolution. Conflict is not necessarily bad for the organization; dealt with properly it can provide the energy to drive the organization forward (Wenzel 1986). On the other hand, conflict without a proper means of resolution can divide the organization and cause it to falter or fail. This is especially true in group practices, where conflict between the physicians will most certainly be present.

Conflict Between Professional and Organization

Conflict between the professional and the organization will always be present and must be understood. Professionals have their own standards, which are often in conflict with those of their organizations. The professional needs freedom, and the organization, in response to complexity, needs processes and procedures by which it can operate. Professionals will generally resist this kind of organizational process; therefore, it is incumbent on the leadership and management to provide an opportunity for the professionals to understand the inner workings of the complex organization and their participation in it. It is doubtful that either the professionals or organizations can be changed; therefore, understanding is the key (Fogel 1989).

It is important to understand the basics of conflict and be able to identify who on the staff of the organization is most likely to be involved in that conflict. Conflict may be between the physician and:

- leadership;
- management;
- other physicians in the group;
- patient; or
- any of the external organizations and individuals that serve the medical practice, including lawyers, accountants, and consultants.

The Resolution Process

The organization's process for conflict resolution should be established long before a significant situation involving conflict arises between any of the parties listed above. That process can begin by bringing the parties involved in the conflict together and moving them to an understanding of what the conflict is really about. Then, help them establish an appropriate resolution mechanism so that they can move from being part of the problem to becoming the solution. For clinical situations the medical director has significant responsibility. When managerial conflicts exist between members of the physician staff and management, the president of the clinic must become involved. The manager, most frequently a nonphysician, should not attempt this resolution process alone because that will only lead to further escalation of the conflict situation.

Conflict can provide the energy necessary for an organization to move forward. At the same time conflict unchecked by a resolution process and allowed to grow can have a profoundly negative effect. It is management's job to resolve these conflicts and use the energy from them to increase the opportunities for the success of the organization.

Summary

This chapter defines the different organizational models found in physician group practices. Physicians and managers should be sure the model they have adopted fits the function of the group. Professional organizations are unique, and leaders and managers must understand their unique attributes.

Over the past 25 years significant legislation and regulation have affected group practice. Changes at both the federal and state levels will continue to have a significant effect on the function and operation of group practice.

There is a strong relationship among the structure of the organization, legal constraints under which it operates its culture, and conflict that can provide energy for growth or paralyze its activities. How these relationships are developed and how the leaders and managers exert their influence will make the difference. The organization and its leadership must have clear focus embedded in strong ideals. A strong leader teamed with a competent manager and an outstanding staff will se the tone for the entire organization.

Discussion Questions

1. Why are the organizational models important, and how do they influence the functions of the group?
2. How have legislation and regulation affected group practice?
3. What are the principal reasons for professional liability suits?

4. What is the relationship between organizational culture and the group's ability to initiate a change process?
5. What is the best approach to conflict resolution?

References

Fogel, D. S. 1989. "The Uniqueness of a Professionally Dominated Organization." *Health Care Management Review* 14 (3): 15–24.

Harris, D. M. 2003. *Contemporary Issues in Healthcare Law and Ethics, 2nd Edition*. Chicago: Health Administration Press.

Showalter, J. S. 2003. *The Law of Healthcare Administration*. Chicago: Health Administration Press.

Wenzel, F. J. 1986. "Conflict: An Imperative for Success." *Journal of Medical Practice Management* 1 (4): 252–59.

———. 1989. "Corporate Culture: The Silent Governor." *Medical Group Management Journal* 36 (3): 33–42.

4

STRATEGIC PLANNING AND MARKETING

Frederick J. Wenzel

Learning Objectives

This chapter will enable the reader to:

- understand the importance of the strategic and marketing planning processes;
- understand the relationship between vision, mission, strategy, and business plans;
- appreciate the need for internal and external research and the evaluation of the strengths, weaknesses, opportunities, and threats to the organization;
- understand the value of market research;
- prepare both strategic and marketing plans for a group practice;
- develop a business plan; and
- develop a plan for evaluating the strategic and marketing plans.

Chapter Purpose

This chapter describes the role of planning in group practice. It provides an understanding of the definitions of vision, mission, strategies, and business plans. Planning begins with a good foundation in both internal and external research as defined by the strengths, weaknesses, opportunities, and threats to the organization. The chapter stresses engaging the members of the group, especially the physicians who need to carry out the plan in the short- and long-term planning process. The annual process, including the time required to create, execute, and evaluate the plan, is described, as is the potential role of consultants. The work or business plan, which identifies individual projects in line with objectives, and a time schedule and person responsible for each task should be committed to paper. Marketing the medical group practice is considered in the light of the strategic plan. The importance of market research along with the methods for evaluating the needs and wants of the customer and the medical group's marketplace through surveys, focus groups, and other methods are described. Market segmentation and marketing mix are also discussed.

Case in Point

Dr. Williams, the president of Merryville multispecialty clinic was meeting with the executive committee to discuss the planning and marketing activities of the organization. He began by asking his colleagues what they understood about the planning process, and the response he received was quite appropriate as the executive committee members outlined their definitions for vision, mission, and strategy. The president was satisfied they understood in sufficient detail that he could begin talking about how they would proceed with the strategic planning process at the retreat scheduled for the following month.

Then he asked a question about their understanding of marketing, and the committee members' unanimous opinion was that marketing was advertising. The president knew immediately he had a great deal of work to do to promote an understanding of what marketing was really all about. Because the marketing plan had to fit with the strategic plan, he believed it was necessary for the planning group to have background information on the definition, purposes, and opportunities of marketing. He asked the administration to provide information on the definition of marketing, market research, marketing planning, implementation, and evaluation. What kinds of data should the administrative staff provide to help the executive committee understand the implications of these topics for the strategic planning process?

Strategic Positioning of the Organization

Role of Strategic Planning and Marketing

Strategic planning and marketing are key elements contributing to the success of a group practice. All organizations must have an idea of where they are going and what they intend to do. Without these critical elements the organization simply proceeds on a random path, conducting its business on a day-to-day basis without discussion. There is little rationale for the way things are done, resulting in missed opportunities and, not infrequently, business failures.

If an organization is to be successful, it must commit itself to both strategic and marketing planning. It is necessary for the group practice to evaluate its market and make decisions about the needs and wants of those they wish to serve. The marketing plan defines which services are to be provided and specifically addresses the issues of place, price, product, and promotion. Organizations that do not pursue a logical plan often find themselves struggling to keep their patient base while confusion reigns about the group's central purpose.

Leadership and Decision Process Issues

Leadership is an essential element in the development of the strategic and marketing plans. Under the direction of the physician president and the chief administrative officer, the organization should have a decision process through which it determines where it wishes to go, what it wishes to become, and what it wishes to do. Without strong leadership at the top of the organization, both the planning and decision processes are doomed to failure. The president must take a lead role as she and the chief administrative officer proceed through the planning process with the board of directors or executive committee.

Frequently the group practice will appoint a special planning group that has not only members of the executive committee or board of directors but other individuals from the group who can make critical contributions to the process. It is better to be inclusive rather than exclusive. All the members of the planning group should know and understand the process to be used for both strategic and market planning. Therefore, it may be necessary to conduct special education programs before the actual planning process is begun.

The definitions used in the planning process should be agreed upon. It is also essential that the decision process be decided upon so the work of the planning group can proceed without constantly reinventing it. A process can be established in which small groups are assigned a certain issue or issues and they are responsible for making recommendations to the main body for review, consideration, and decision. This calls for a structured presentation, discussion, and voting process. When this is in place and the pre-planning work is completed, it will be necessary in most cases to take the final plan recommendations to the board and the membership at large for their endorsement.

The Fraternity Versus the Group

Many group practices, especially those that are new or growing rapidly, are much more like fraternities than group practices. Everyone is for themselves, and the organization is low on the list of priorities. For an organization to achieve success and longevity it must move from the fraternity attitude to a marketing and business orientation (Rubin and Fernandez 1991). If the organization is to achieve great success it must move to a stage of organizational actualization.

In order for the practice to be a real group each individual must give up some autonomy in the interest of the organization. For most physicians this is not too difficult, but some simply do not fit into a group practice and are much better off practicing on their own. A great deal of time can be consumed trying to deal with outliers. When physicians are recruited to the group these issues should be discussed in detail, and the culture and goals of the organization should be understood by everyone. If this educational process is done properly and effectively, the organization will be cohesive and the planning process will be a much easier task. There is little or no room for the fraternity concept in group practice.

The Actualized Group

It is difficult to define an actualized group, but when a group has reached this stage of organizational evolution it is quite apparent. The members of the organization have a clear vision of where the organization is headed, and they have a clear understanding of the group's mission. The focus is on the patient. The relationship between the physicians is collegial; they know and understand they are in the practice together. The organization is the vehicle through which they can accomplish the central purpose of delivering high-quality medical care. Service to the organization and the patient is a key element that strengthens the foundation of the group practice.

Definitions and Steps in Group Practice Planning

SWOT Analysis

Before an organization begins the planning process it should undertake an evaluation of both the internal and external environments by observing the organization's strengths, weaknesses, opportunities, and threats (SWOT). The organization's strengths (a culture that embraces change) and weaknesses (a disproportionately large overhead) must be acknowledged and honestly stated. Most organizations have opportunities they have never considered. For instance, the clinic was offered an opportunity for a joint venture, which it turned down. That offer was taken by another group and turned out to be very profitable. The planning process provides a good environment for discovery to take place. Threats, whether internal or external, should also be acknowledged. Often internal threats are overlooked and the plans, no matter how well conceived, can be subverted from within the organization, such as a lukewarm adoption made by middle management. The information should be gathered as widely as possible and be completely objective. Some organizations use a consultant to conduct this aspect of the planning process to promote objectivity.

As part of the investigation of the threats, the organization should also carefully evaluate its competition; as the positioning plans are developed. Competitive response is a key factor in any strategic plan, and failure to take it into consideration can lead to significant surprises that can prevent the organization from achieving its stated goals. Some physicians are familiar with this process, but many are not. It is imperative before the planning process begins that all the physicians and senior staff understand the implications of the strengths, weaknesses, opportunities, and threats in both the internal and external environments.

The planning group must understand the relationship of the factors outlined above to the culture of the organization, which in physician groups is different than in a hospital or most other healthcare settings. The professional organization has standards that can often stand in the way of an effective planning process unless they are clearly understood. Planning with professionals is different. Continuing the planning process will be much easier once all of these factors are clearly understood and the organization can begin thinking about its focus and positioning.

In some groups it is best to approach planning incrementally, as proposed by Quinn (1989) in his study of logical incrementalism. Quinn postulated that the best plans with optimal chance for success are done in small steps that follow each other in a logical sequence. In this way small successes accumulate to make big successes. This approach can be helpful to a group as it begins its first plan.

Vision Statement

The vision statement is best defined as an organization's determination of where it wishes to go or what it wishes to be. In the group practice environment the practice might want to be a premier multispecialty organization delivering high-quality care to all who seek care. Or in a single-specialty group the vision statement might say that the organization wishes to be the premier provider of orthopedic services in the region. Even the smallest of physician organizations should have a vision of where they are headed or what they want to be. Without understanding and commitment it is difficult for the organization to sustain itself. The vision statement should be brief, clear, and concise.

Mission Statement

The mission statement describes what the organization will do to realize its vision. The two statements go together, and they are a unifying conceptual framework for what follows in the strategies, goals, and objectives. The mission of the organization may be to practice high-quality medicine and care for patients in a compassionate, effective, and efficient manner. There are a number of variations on this theme, depending on the kind of services delivered. If the organization is involved in research and education, these elements should also be incorporated into the mission. The mission statement should, like the vision, be brief and to the point. If the mission statement says that the organization will serve all who seek care, operationalizing that aspect of the statement should be carefully evaluated in the light of current economic conditions. There may also be differences in the missions of various practice organizations, depending on whether they are for-profit or not-for-profit, academic, or single- or multispecialty.

Strategies

These statements must be tied to and flow out of the mission statement of the organization. They are usually broad and provide the direction to guide the organization and its staff. There may, for instance, be a strategy for recruiting and retaining physicians, a strategy that deals with the financial positioning of the organization, or a strategy to develop a center of excellence. The strategies can be considered essential foundations for the development of the Balanced Scorecard (Kaplan and Norton 1996). The purpose of the Balanced Scorecard is to acknowledge that although financial goals are important, so are quality, patient satisfaction, staff morale, and other aspects of the human side of the enterprise. These strategic statements should be no longer than one or two paragraphs, and they should pave the way for the development of the goals and objectives.

Goals and Objectives

The goals and objectives divide the strategy into a manageable series of elements with increasing focus. A goal statement describes one aspect of the strategy as a manageable activity. For example, a goal related to the recruiting strategy would be to "develop the medical specialties necessary to support a comprehensive cancer program." This goal would have a number of objectives, which would be still more specific and of much shorter term. One objective might be to "hire two oncologists in the next 18 months." Another might be to "hire the complementary nursing staff to support the oncologists." The strategy, goals, and objectives are the roadmap for accomplishing the organization's mission. They serve as the template for evaluation of how well the organization is operationalizing its mission (Andrews 1987). Box 4.1 provides a brief strategic plan.

Business Plan

The business plan consists of a series of short-term objectives identifying what, how, who, when, and where. It can be as simple as a grid with the objectives in the left column and a column for each of the elements to the right. Business plans are usually written for the short term, generally for a period of one year. As an example, the objectives outlined in Box 4.1 could become part of the business plan. That aspect of the plan would identify why the objective should be undertaken, who would carry it out, how it would be accomplished, when it would be accomplished, and how it will be evaluated.

Evaluation of the Strategic Plan

The broad strategic plan should be evaluated on an annual basis, generally just before the annual strategic planning process begins. The exercise is one in which the president or administrator presents the business plan for the preceding year along with an evaluation of how well the organization has done in

VISION	The clinic will be known throughout the region for its outstanding, sophisticated patient care.
MISSION	The clinic will deliver high-quality care, with a focus on service based in research and education, to all who seek that care.
STRATEGY	The principal focus of the clinic will be on timely, sophisticated patient care that will be delivered by caring providers. Access will be stressed, and both effectiveness (quality) and efficiency (cost) will be maintained at all levels of care.
GOAL	All patients will have appropriate access to the care system in a timely fashion.
OBJECTIVES	• Quality of care will be evaluated on a continuing basis in each department under the direction of the medical director.
	• A system of open access will be developed to serve patients on a more timely basis.
	• Nurse triage will be developed to place the patient in the most appropriate environment for their care.
	• Cost of care will be evaluated on a continuing basis using activity-based accounting methods.

BOX 4.1
Abbreviated
Example of a
Strategic Plan

meeting its stated strategies, goals, and objectives. This should be done before more specific plans are laid for the following year. The organization may find itself unable to accomplish some of the goals and objectives outlined and may need to reconsider the strategy. Sometimes it may even be necessary to reconsider the mission. Ordinarily the change will occur in the strategy, and the adoption of a new set of goals and objectives (perhaps a change in direction) will allow the organization to accomplish what it set out to do. Evaluation is a critical aspect of the process.

Planning for Small Physician Groups

Planning for large physician group practices is a difficult task unless there is sufficient staff to support the effort. Planning for small physician groups is even more difficult for reasons beyond staff resources. Often the physicians believe the organization will continue, without giving any thought to a vision, mission, or any type of plan. The belief is that there will always be a sufficient number of patients to be seen. Government regulations, while imposing, can be circumvented because "they don't really apply to us." The plan for the group often resides in the mind of the founder or those physicians who have been with the group for a long time. The trouble generally begins when they hire young associates who have different ideas about how the practice should be conducted. If there has been no plan or planning process in place, the associates wonder whether there is direction and how this will affect their futures.

Small groups can plan effectively, however, and the process can generally be simplified if everyone in the group is involved. Through a facilitated process they can articulate the group's vision and mission and outline a series of goals and objectives they would like to achieve in the next year. This will provide sufficient direction for a small organization as long as an evaluation plan is in place. A qualified consultant is helpful in this process, in which learning accompanies the planning.

Marketing in Group Practice

Marketing Defined

Berkowitz (1996, p. 6) defined marketing as the "analysis, planning, implementation, and control of carefully formulated programs designed to bring about voluntary exchanges of values with target markets for the purpose of achieving organizational objectives." He also stated that, "Central to the definition of marketing is the focus on the consumer, whether that be an individual patient, physician, or organization, such as a company contracting for industrial medicine" (Berkowitz 1996, p. 4).

Berkowitz's definition can appropriately be applied to physician group practices. First it emphasizes that these organizations should pay attention to the four Ps of marketing—product (service), price, place, and promotion—described by McCarthy in 1960. In order to be successful, group practices must have a marketing orientation, which is best described above. In the exchange of values the physician organization is on one side and the patients, referring physicians, payers, hospitals, and all other organizations with which the group is involved are on the other. They are the customers and the target populations to be served. Unfortunately most physicians and administrators define marketing as advertising and let it go at that, missing the point of a marketing orientation completely.

The foundation of a good marketing plan is market research (Grapentine 1998). The organization has to determine what populations it wishes to serve and then evaluate or assess that population to evaluate its needs and desires (Berkowitz 1996). If the population is broad, it may be necessary to segment and focus the market research on a specific group. After the evaluation is complete the organization should look at its resources and abilities to deliver the needed or desired services. The next focus should be on pricing (paying attention to the competition) and the place these services are to be delivered under optimal circumstances. Next a promotional program should be put in place to inform the target markets of the availability of the services. An evaluation plan should also be formulated to determine whether

A marketing research study conducted in an upper-middle-class area of the community showed a potential opportunity for the clinic to develop a healthy lifestyles program. The competition appeared modest, so the clinic developed a comprehensive program of services and a marketing promotion to educate the community about the program. An evaluation plan was also developed, then conducted on a quarterly basis. It included the number of new individuals using the service, number of times the individual used the service, types of services used, and customer satisfaction with the services offered. The demographics of the users were also studied to ensure the facilities were meeting the needs of the various groups.

BOX 4.2
Example of a
Marketing
Evaluation
Plan

the marketing effort and provision of the services have been successful. Box 4.2 provides an example of such an evaluation.

Marketing Perspective and Orientation

The group practice manager must pay a great deal of attention to the perspective of marketing inside the organization if it is to be successful. It is simple to say, "If we build it they will come," but this belief does not lead to growth and success in group practice. The first and perhaps most important duty the manager has is to convince the physicians that marketing is not simply advertising, but rather an orientation for the entire organization that begins with market research and understanding the needs of the population to be served. When group practices first started, it was sufficient to be an inside-out organization, but in the current competitive environment this model no longer holds; all group practices must become outside-in organizations. In other words, they set out to determine the needs of those they wish to serve and then develop the resources to provide those services to the identified populations effectively and efficiently.

Internal and External Marketing

The manager must pay attention to two important publics—the internal and external markets—when considering a marketing orientation. Each of these markets has distinct needs. If an organization is viewed from the marketing perspective, the staff, especially those who provide hands-on medical care, are part of the marketing staff. The impression patients have of the clinic and its services is a result of the treatment they receive from the staff. Therefore, it is important that all staff members are trained in customer relations.

Fottler, Ford, and Heaton's (2002) notion of "healing hospitality" has great merit and validity. The satisfied patient is one of the best promotional tools a clinic can have. That patient tells friends and relatives about the great services he received. On the other hand an unhappy patient tells everyone he encounters about the poor services and his dissatisfaction. The result is obvious. Quality in the eyes of patients is largely connected with the way they were treated by the staff.

External marketing should play a major role in all organizations; as discussed above efforts should begin with marketing research and move quickly to market planning and implementation of the services deemed necessary to meet the needs and wants of those to be served. While great attention should be paid to the patient, attention must also be paid to the referring physicians. They are an important source of patients, especially for specialty services, and they must be treated with consideration. One of the best ways of building strong relationships with referring physicians is to call them about their patients as soon as possible and be sure that the patients return to their care.

The marketing plan must take into consideration the resources needed to provide new services as well as the competition, which will quickly take note of any new service offerings. The competition should be evaluated carefully, and the organization should not be surprised if competitors respond by offering a similar service; the group should instead be prepared to respond in a rational fashion.

Market Research

Depending on the size of the organization marketing research can be done by in-house staff or consultants. It is important that this research be conducted by individuals skilled in market research because this science has become sophisticated and requires special expertise. A number of healthcare consulting firms have strong market research credentials. If the manager is considering bringing one of these consultant groups on board, she should review its members' credentials carefully. The manager should contact previous clients to determine the degree of satisfaction with the consulting services. It will be necessary for the organization to outline its marketing objectives clearly before the consultation begins. A contract with the marketing firm should also clearly spell out the consulting deliverables. The work of the consultant should be evaluated on a periodic basis so there will be no surprises.

Evaluation of Marketing Activities

The results of all of the marketing activities should be evaluated on a periodic basis. This can be accomplished in a variety of ways. The manager should pay attention to the four Ps of marketing while conducting these evaluations. If part of the marketing plan is place, the location should be evaluated for fit with the patient population. The ambience of the facility should also be evaluated on a periodic basis. If price is a principal consideration, this should be tested as well. The manager should be cautious about comparing prices with other organizations, however, because of antitrust price-fixing regulations. Product or service should also be evaluated carefully; if the marketing plan is functioning properly, the number of services being requested by the target market will increase. Finally all promotional activities ought to be evaluated on a periodic basis. Often organizations advertise in various media such as newspaper and phone book ads. Seldom, however, is an evaluation conducted to determine whether the advertising is really effective. Such advertising can be expensive, and the manager must pay attention to these costs. On a final note about promotion, we should remember the staff when it comes to these activities. They are an important part of the marketing effort; when they have done a good job, they should be rewarded.

Summary

This chapter describes the strategic and marketing planning processes for physician group practices. Several important elements must be in place to ensure success: strong support from the leadership of the group, careful SWOT analysis, good market research, attention to the four Ps of marketing, and sound evaluation process. The other most important consideration is involvement of the physician members of the group and the management staff. Buy-in by the majority of the physicians is critical.

Discussion Questions

1. Why is planning sometimes difficult in the group practice setting?
2. How can the administrator help facilitate the planning process?
3. Why is it important to prepare an annual business plan?
4. Is marketing simply advertising?
5. Describe the importance of market research.
6. Which of the four Ps do you think is the most important?

References

Andrews, K. R. 1987. *The Concept of Corporate Strategy, 3rd Edition*. Homewood, IL: R. D. Irwin.

Berkowitz, E. N. 1996. *Essentials of Healthcare Marketing*. Gaithersburg, MD: Aspen Publishers.

Fottler, M. D., R. C. Ford, and C. Heaton. 2002. *Achieving Service Excellence*. Chicago: Health Administration Press.

Grapentine, T. 1998. "Practical Theory." *Marketing Research*. 10 (2): 4–12.

Kaplan, R. S., and D. P. Norton. 1996. "Using the Balanced Scorecard as a Strategic Management System." *Harvard Business Review*. 74 (1): 75–85.

McCarthy, E. J. 1960. *Basic Marketing: A Managerial Approach.* Homewood, IL: R. D. Irwin

Quinn, J. B. 1989. "Strategic Change: 'Logical Incrementalism.'" *Sloan Management Review* 30 (4): 45–60.

Fernandez, C.R., and I.M. Rubin (Eds.). 1991. *My Pulse Is Not What It Used to Be: The Leadership Challenges in Healthcare.* Honolulu: The Temenos Foundation.

FINANCIAL MANAGEMENT

Joseph P. White

Learning Objectives

This chapter will enable the reader to:

- understand the uniqueness of accounting and finance for medical groups;
- explain the different reimbursement methods;
- grasp resource-based relative values and fee schedules;
- build a budget for a medical group;
- understand the different valuation methods in addition to liquidity, solvency, and profitability ratios for medical groups;
- determine why medical groups choose different types of entities from a tax perspective; and
- understand some of the differences in retirement plans and their importance in medical groups.

Chapter Purpose

This chapter provides the reader with the basic principles of finance as they relate to the unique characteristics of medical groups. Financial management has as its foundation both financial and managerial accounting; readers are assumed to have a basic understanding of both. The chapter describes the financial management of the group practice organization introduced in earlier chapters. Areas considered include budgeting, valuation, financial ratios, and retirement plans; each specific (and sometimes unique) to the not-for-profit or for-profit group practice organization.

Case in Point

Dr. Williams was puzzling over the new financial statements. He called the chief financial officer (CFO) and the administrator to discuss the composition of the financial reports and how they might be best explained both to

the board of directors and the membership of the group at large. The CFO pointed out that accounting statements "are what they are" and should be easily understood by the physicians. The administrator, however, suggested that few physicians have a financial background, making it difficult for them to understand the financial status of the clinic given the complexity of the financial statements. He emphasized that most of the physicians did not understand the difference between cash and accrual accounting and because the clinic is on an accrual system, that would have to be explained carefully.

Dr. Williams suggested that the two staff members get together and develop a reporting system that could be understood, with some coaching, by most of the members of the staff. He also suggested that management consider a financial seminar for the physicians that would include the reading and interpretation of financial statements. He stressed that it would be important for the physicians to understand how the financial status of the organization affected the physician compensation system. The administrator and CFO went to work. What would be a good starting point in their efforts to help physicians understand the group's financial picture?

Historical Perspective of Accounting and Finance for Medical Groups

Physicians and their respective medical groups have a tremendous influence on the economic success of healthcare institutions. A hospital cannot be successful if it does not have physicians providing services. A financially successful medical group in a community does not guarantee a successful hospital, but a financially suffering medical staff is definitely a cause for concern. The economic interdependence between the hospital and the medical group led to the consolidation of many primary care groups (family practice, internal medicine, pediatrics, and obstetrics and gynecology) in the early 1990s (Coddington 2001).

An understanding of medical group finance, economics, and accounting is critical to understanding healthcare finance. Because they are most often the entry point into the healthcare system, physicians comprise an integral component of the organization's financial status.

Cash Basis Versus Accrual Basis

Many medical groups operate on a modified cash basis of accounting as opposed to the accrual method. The cash basis recognizes revenue when payment is received and records expenses when paid. The accrual method recognizes revenue when earned and records expenses when incurred. The cash basis is an industry standard, but it is being replaced with the more traditional accrual method as groups grow larger. The large number of medical groups

that have been acquired by hospital systems usually switch to an accrual method.

The cash basis standard most likely had its roots in small medical practices and sole proprietorships. Such organizations found the cash basis financial system easier to produce and understand. Practices most likely reported their income taxes on a cash basis and did not want to have two sets of books—cash basis for tax reporting and accrual for management reporting.

The physician is often involved with the billing and accounts payable functions in small practices. Historically physicians had little need to have their financial statements provided to bankers or other outside practices. They knew in detail what was going on in their businesses on a day-to-day basis through the practice's checkbook.

In a solo practice the physician paid all the bills, and what was left in the checkbook was his compensation. In many ways this holds true today; in independent medical groups the year-end bonus is paid out based on how much cash is available and the level of taxable income before the bonus is paid out.

Financial Reporting Needs

Financial reporting for medical groups can be more complicated than in other businesses. Most businesses have financial reporting needs related to income tax, stakeholder, and management purposes. Medical groups often have an additional reporting need related to physician compensation or income distribution formula.

Tax Reporting

Independent medical groups tend to report income tax returns on an income tax or modified cash basis ("modified" because equipment is capitalized and depreciated over time and retirement plan contributions are recorded in the year in which the expense is incurred as opposed to when paid).

Some medical groups are required to keep some of their business lines on the accrual basis of accounting for income tax purposes. Examples include ophthalmology practices that own optical dispensaries. Because the optical division sells eyewear and maintains an inventory of eye glasses, it is required to report that portion of the business on the accrual basis.

Many of the largest medical groups (e.g., Mayo Clinic, Cleveland Clinic, Park Nicollet, Marshfield Clinic) in the United States are not-for-profit corporations under section 501(c)(3) of the IRS code. These organizations do not pay income taxes on revenues in excess of their expenses (note that we avoid the word "profits") from business lines related to providing healthcare to patients. Tax reporting in not-for-profits is different than that in for-profit medical groups. The reporting is no less complicated, but the motivation of for-profit medical groups to avoid paying income taxes unnecessarily is strong.

Stakeholder Reporting

Stakeholder reporting in for-profit medical groups includes physician shareholders, lenders, and other creditors. The reporting usually consists of year-end financial statements prepared by an outside public accounting firm, which could audit, review, or compile the financials. The level of service provided by the accounting firm is often related to the size of the group. Smaller groups (ten physicians or fewer) tend to have compiled financials, and larger groups tend to have reviewed and audited financial statements. Sample financial reports are included in Appendix 5.1.

Management Purposes

Management reporting for medical groups should include the traditional financial statements (balance sheet, income statement, and statement of cash flows) on a monthly basis along with several dashboard indicators designed for that practice. Included in these should be:

- Accounts receivable
  —Number of days outstanding
  —Aging by payer
- Overhead as a percentage of revenue
- Relative value units (RVUs) produced in total and by provider and location
- Receipts or revenue per RVU
- Total overhead expenses per RVU
- Subcategories of overhead per RVU
  —Human resource expense
    - Administrative
    - Business office
    - Nursing (RN, LPN, medical assistants)

In each specialty additional ratios will be critical to the success of the practice's performance measurement and search for trends. Examples include number of scans done in an imaging center and new patients for pediatrics. Sample management reports are included in Appendix 5.2.

Income Distribution Formulas

As the old saying goes, "Money makes the world go 'round." A physician practice, like any business, must competitively compensate its employees or it will cease to exist. A physician may make $100,000 or $500,000 depending on the specialty, but if compensation is significantly higher in a practice across town or across the country, it will be difficult if not impossible for the lower-compensating practice to survive in the long run. This leads to significant time and money (internal staff time and outside consultants) spent on calculating and searching for the perfect methodology or formula. While many professional service organizations (lawyers, engineers, and so on) focus on compensation formulas, the medical community has created an entire industry around it.

Larger healthcare systems and physician groups have shifted away from complex formulas to payment on a per-RVU basis. Several organizations provide survey data on compensation, including the Medical Group Management Association (MGMA) and American Medical Group Association (AMGA). These surveys are widely used to help determine market compensation; however, caution should be used as markets can change quickly and surveys can be biased or yield inaccurate data.

Most independent for-profit medical groups pay all nonphysician expenses (overhead), then split the net income. This method ensures that the group cannot overpay physicians.

Compensation programs are far from an exact science, and it seems that for every different group there is a different method. However, there are some common methods (see Appendix 5.3):

- 100 percent productivity based
- Allocation of revenue and expenses
- Splitting net income, from 100 percent equal to a small amount equally divided among the groups physicians and the remainder based on production

The different methods tell a great deal about the culture of the group. Groups that share a large amount of income equally may find themselves with productivity problems. This means that physicians do not see the number of patients per day that their peers in other groups see, leading to less revenue and thus less profit to be shared among the physicians. A group that has a highly productivity-based compensation method may find the physicians competing for patients within the group. This type of behavior makes it difficult to build a strong team culture.

There is no magic formula for the payment of physician services. Physicians are reluctant to trust a compensation system that allocates income based on subjective criteria such as patient satisfaction or utilization. Their scientific training may cause the majority of physicians to search for a method that is fair to all parties. Unfortunately the best formula might be one in which every one is equally unhappy.

Compensation Methods and the Stark Law

In 1995 the federal self-referral law went into effect. Commonly know as the Stark Law, it prohibits physicians from receiving direct compensation for ancillary services (laboratory services, x-ray, and other services). This had the effect of requiring physicians to change compensation methods to disallow receipt of production credit for laboratory services and x-rays ordered.

The Stark Law has had a significant impact on the healthcare industry and is extremely complex; Chapter 3 discusses it in greater detail. While the laws include services covered only by Medicare and Medicaid, most groups find it easier to treat all insurance payers alike and do not differentiate between them.

Chart of Accounts

A chart of accounts is a system of laying out a group's assets, liabilities, revenues, and expenses. It is the nuts and bolts of building the general ledger system and the financial statements of any business.

MGMA (Piland and Glass 1999) published a chart of accounts for healthcare organizations. It is recommended that medical groups use this format for the basis of producing financial statements. The consistent chart of accounts allows groups to produce financial statements in a consistent format and make comparisons between groups.

Organizational Structure of Medical Groups

Most independent medical groups are organized as professional associations (PAs). As discussed in Chapter 3, professional corporations are corporations and limited liability companies (LLCs) organized for the purpose of providing professional services. A professional limited liability partnership (PLLP) is the partnership equivalent. Shareholders or partners of a professional organization must be professionals (physicians in this case). In some states midlevel providers are allowed to be members of a professional service organization. What services constitute professional services are defined by state law and differ from state to state.

Some of these laws have the effect of making it illegal for hospitals or publicly held corporations to own physician practices. The intent of this type of law is to have professionals involved in decision making to ensure that quality is in the hands of those who can effectively judge it.

Hospitals and publicly held corporations have circumvented this requirement by establishing management service organizations that own all the assets of the physician organization and then enter into a long-term agreement (a professional service agreement) with the physician group to provide medical services. The benefit of being a professional corporation or PLLP is the assurance that a professional will be in the position of making decisions related to medical issues.

What Makes Healthcare Finance Unique?

The reimbursement methods used to pay physicians for the services they provide are what make healthcare finance truly unique. Understanding these reimbursement methods is necessary to gain a complete picture of how a medical group works.

Current Procedural Terminology (CPT) Codes

All procedures related to patient care that a physician performs have been assigned a *Current Procedural Terminology (CPT®)* code, which was developed by the American Medical Association (AMA 2002) to provide healthcare professionals with a uniform language for effective communication. The CPT codes are continually reviewed, revised, and updated to reflect changes in medical care.

Coding is complex because of the large number of codes and the decisions related to when to use a certain code as opposed to another. Coding is critical from a financial perspective because the physician or coder bases reimbursement on the CPT code that has been assigned. Many organizations employ certified coders who assign codes based on physician notes and dictation. Figure 5.1 shows some examples of coding questions.

Consultations

A physician in our practice referred his patient to a specialist within our group for treatment of his arthritis. Can the specialist charge a consultation for this visit?

The terms "consultation" and "referral" are confusing to many providers. A consultation is performed when a patient (new or established) is seen by a physician whose opinion or advice is sought by another physician. The consulting physician must report his findings to the requesting physician. In this case, as the diagnosis is known and no opinion is being sought, no consultation can be coded.

So what does the physician charge? The correct code for this visit would be the appropriate level of evaluation and management (E/M) service (established patient or new patient if not seen by this specialist within the last three years).

New Patient Versus Established Patient

Two years ago a patient was seen by a cardiologist who has since left our practice. The patient was seen today by our gastroenterology specialist for a new problem. Do we charge a new or established patient E/M service?

CPT definition of a new patient is one who has not received professional services from the physician, or another physician of the same specialty who belongs to the group practice, within the last three years. As the physicians in this case have two different specialties, the appropriate new patient E/M can be charged.

[Note: The new patient charge is reimbursed at a higher rate.]

Lesion Removal

Our physician removed a 1-cm lesion from a patient's arm and sent the specimen for pathology. Can we charge for the removal and for the biopsy?

When removing a lesion from a patient, obtaining a tissue specimen is a routine component of the procedure. The biopsy is considered incidental to the procedure and not separately reportable.

[Note: Charging for the biopsy would be an example of improper coding. The federal fines for improper coding are extreme, and physicians can be sentenced to prison time for fraudulent coding.]

FIGURE 5.1
Examples of Coding Questions

Resource-based Relative Value Scale (RBRVS)

In 1992 Medicare changed the way it reimbursed physicians for the services provided. In the past reimbursement was based on gross charges. Medical groups submitted bills to Medicare, and Medicare paid an amount known as "usual and customary." Usual and customary was based on the average (or some percentage of the average) of the charges that had been submitted to Medicare. The government standardized the way it pays for physician services by implementing a fee schedule based on a resource-based relative value scale (RBRVS). The values were assigned as part of a Harvard study (Hsiao et al. 1992) commissioned by the Centers for Medicare & Medicaid Services, formerly known as the Health Care Financing Administration.

RBRVS assigned a value to each CPT code. The value was based on three components: physician work, practice expense, and malpractice insurance expense. The physician work component was designed to take into account cognitive skill required, time to complete the procedure, skill required, education, stress associated with the procedure, and risk to the patient. The practice expense and malpractice expense components were designed to cover the overhead or operating costs of a practice and the professional liability insurance expense. Each of the three components is then adjusted by a geographic factor to reflect that the resource cost can be different in different regions of the country (see Tables 5.1 and 5.2).

Medicare sets a conversion factor each year based on budgeted Medicare dollars available and expected utilization in the coming year. For

TABLE 5.1
Established Patient Office Visit (in Minnesota; CPT Code 99213)

	RVU	Geographic Practice Cost Indices	Product
Professional Work RVU	.67	.990	.66
Practice Expense RVU	.43	.966	.42
Malpractice Cost RVU	.03	.551	.02
Total RVU	1.13		1.10

TABLE 5.2
Coronary Artery Bypass (in Minnesota; CPT Code 33510)

	RVU	Geographic Practice Cost Indices	Product
Professional Work RVU	25.12	.990	24.87
Practice Expense RVU	27.63	.966	26.69
Malpractice Cost RVU	5.20	.551	2.87
Total RVU	57.95		54.42

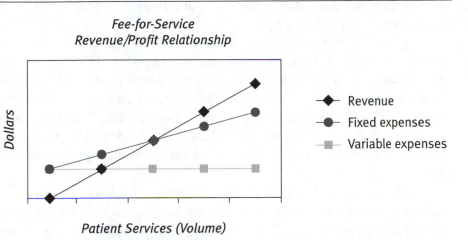

Fee-for-Service Revenue/Profit Relationship

- ◆ Revenue
- ● Fixed expenses
- ▪ Variable expenses

Dollars

Patient Services (Volume)

FIGURE 5.2

Fee-for-service and Discounted Fee-for-service

2004 the conversion factor was $37.3374 and increased 1.5 percent (the minimum increase currently allowed) for 2005.

From Tables 5.1 and 5.2 it is apparent that the geographic adjustment factor decreases the total RVU assigned to these CPT codes for the Minnesota region. This decreases the reimbursement from Medicare because the conversion factor is multiplied by the product to obtain the reimbursement rate. An example of the 2004 Geographic Practice Cost Indices can be found in Appendix 5.4.

Fee-for-service and Discounted Fee-for-service

In a fee-for-service system the more services provided by a medical group, the greater the revenue earned (see Figure 5.2). Once a medical group covers its fixed expenses and variable costs it begins to make a profit. This allows a medical group to make a profit on additional services as long as it is covering the variable costs.

This revenue-profit relationship was one factor that led some groups to accept discounts from third-party payers. Groups were willing (or needed) to accept less than their standard fee schedule in order to be preferred providers. A preferred provider is a physician who accepts an insurance company's payment while other providers do not (meaning that a patient may need to pay more for the services of a provider who does not have preferred status with the patient's insurance company). In theory by accepting a discount the medical group is hoping to attract more patients and provide more services.

Most groups now set their fee schedules by multiplying the RVUs (before geographic adjustments) assigned to a CPT code by a conversion factor for a group of CPT codes. For example, a conversion factor of $65 will set all evaluation and management code fees, and surgical code fees will be set using a conversion factor of $85.

In the healthcare world fee schedules can be set at any level; however, insurance companies, health maintenance organizations (HMOs), and the government will pay based on the rates contracted with them or what is billed them—whichever is lower. So naturally medical practices tend to inflate their fee schedules to ensure that money is not "left on the table." This has led to discounts being a normal part of medical practice operations. Figure 5.3 demonstrates what has happened to collections in medical groups over the years.

These decreased collections are a reflection of fee schedule increases and reimbursement decreases (or at least not keeping up with the fee schedule increases) from HMOs. The gross collection percentage is the average amount collected compared to what is billed. The adjusted collection percentage is the percentage collected compared to the contracted amount.

Fee schedule development and analysis might look like Table 5.3. An analysis often compares the reimbursement per RVU.

FIGURE 5.3
Relationship Between Adjusted and Gross Collections Over Time

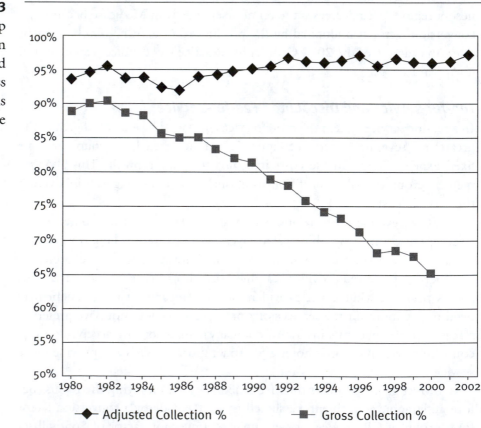

Procedure Code	Current Fee	Medicare Fee	Major Insurance Company	Medicaid Fee	Workers' Comp Fee	% of Total	RVUs
33510	$3,477.00	$1920.96	$2,098.65	$2,341.25	$3,446.29	2%	57.95
76090	$ 107.40	$ 60.83	$ 66.46	$ 41.25	$ 106.45	9%	1.79
76604	$ 130.20	$ 73.90	$ 80.74	$ 168.75	$ 129.05	3%	2.17
92014	$ 99.60	$ 46.61	$ 50.92	$ 27.75	$ 98.72	2%	1.66
92213	$ 67.80	$ 38.16	$ 41.69	$ 24.00	$ 67.20	15%	1.13
99241	$ 81.60	$ 34.27	$ 37.44	$ 45.00	$ 80.88	6%	1.36

TABLE 5.3
Fee Schedule Development and Analysis

Capitation

Capitation is a method of payment in which the third-party payer (an insurance company or HMO) pays the provider group a set rate per member per month for a specific set of medical services. Full-risk capitation means that the provider is taking all the risk associated with an individual patient for healthcare expenditures related to the individual. These include everything from office visits to transplants and premature deliveries. This method of payment was popular in the 1980s and early 1990s, but it is for the most part limited to California at this time.

Figure 5.4 represents the revenue-expense relationship in a capitated environment. The more services provided, the less the group makes.

The thought was that capitation would help physicians control the cost of medical care and discourage the ordering of unnecessary procedures or tests for the sake of additional revenue. The concern associated with this method of reimbursement is that it may provide an incentive to withhold medical care. Some say this method of payment puts the physician at odds with the patient.

Budgeting and Budget Planning and Evaluation

Budgeting should be based on the strategic plan and goals for an organization. A budget should reflect the goals and objectives and the organizational mission and strategies. Most often these are broken into operational and capital budgets.

Annual Operating Budget

As with any business a budget can be a valuable tool for healthcare managers. A sophisticated budgeting process begins by estimating revenue and determining the profit required to fund future growth and capital needs. The

FIGURE 5.4
Revenue-
expense
Relationships in
a Capitated
Environment

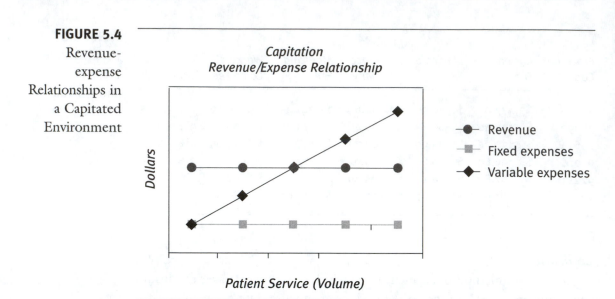

budget should then determine the costs and expenses required to meet the needs of the organization within the budget parameters.

The process should not be to estimate revenue, subtract estimated expenses, and accept the results. Larger healthcare systems budget for a profit in the range of 2 percent to 4 percent of net revenue each year. Smaller medical groups tend to not budget at all; if they do, they budget with the assumption that all profits will be distributed to the shareholders as bonuses. As groups develop and grow they often begin to recognize the benefit of retaining profit for future capital needs and growth.

Revenue Estimation:
Provider productivity

Determining the amount of revenue a medical group will earn begins with a process of listing all providers who bill for procedures and what the individuals have produced in terms of gross charges, number of patient visits, and RVUs. A good process is to provide the historical data to the individual providers and ask for their input on what they think their individual production will be. Many medical groups pay providers based on production, so the process tends to be fairly accurate.

For new providers without historical data an estimate of production can be arrived at by comparison to other providers as they began practices or by comparison to benchmark data. (MGMA is an excellent source of productivity data.) It usually takes about 18 months for a new provider to reach full capacity.

Types of procedures

The organization should take into account any changes in the types of procedures that may occur from one year to the next. Such shifts could result from a change in providers' coding patterns as they receive education related to coding. For example, based on additional documentation in the medical record a group finds that it can code some visits that had been coded as CPT code 99213 as 99214. This will result in greater charges and RVUs and thus greater revenue for the medical group.

A change could be the result of new providers (e.g., specialists), services (e.g., heart scans), or equipment (e.g., CT or MRI machines). The revenue associated with the new services should be known because of the estimates done when the equipment purchase or project assessment was being considered.

Once a group projects the number of RVUs that will be produced, it should determine if the organization's payer mix will change. The payer mix lists the percentage of charges made to each of the principal payers. For example, Table 5.4 represents the percentage of all charges billed to the various insurance carriers and private payers with which a group contracts.

Payer mix

A shift in the payer mix to a greater Medicare percentage and a lower commercial third-party payer can mean a shift in revenue. If Medicare reimburses the medical group in Table 5.4 less than does United Health Care, the group will receive less revenue even if it produces the same number of RVUs.

The medical group should track the payer mix percentages quarterly and have an understanding of which third-party payers are gaining or losing market share. This tracking will not only affect budgeting but may also be necessary for contracting purposes. It should help to identify the good and bad payers.

Cost shifting occurs when the cost of providing care to one group of patients is not covered by the reimbursement levels received from their insurance companies. For years the cost of care for Medicare and Medicaid patients exceeded the reimbursement level. In order to continue to provide care to these patients, providers had to charge other payers at higher levels, hence the term "cost shifting" (see Figure 5.5).

Cost shifting

Payer	2001	2002	2003	2004	2005 Projected
Medicare	30%	32%	35%	36%	38%
Medicaid	10%	10%	11%	11%	11%
BlueCross	33%	28%	30%	29%	29%
United Health Care	27%	21%	16%	17%	15%
Commercial Insurer	5%	5%	5%	5%	5%
Private Pay	5%	4%	3%	2%	2%
Total	100%	100%	100%	100%	100%

TABLE 5.4
Sample Payer Mix

FIGURE 5.5

Cost Shifting

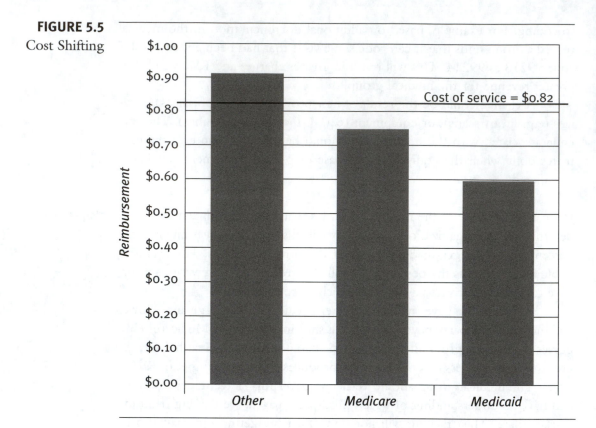

The shifting of costs to commercial insurers and the employers who pay for the majority of the premiums is one reason insurance premiums are expensive.

Expense estimation   The budgeting process requires that expenses match the revenue estimates and profit requirements. A good budget starts with a zero base and does not simply build on the previous year's expenses. Factors to be considered include:

- number of physicians and clinic professionals (providers);
- compensation for each provider;
- salary changes;
- number of support staff and compensation changes;
- changes in benefit costs (e.g., pension, FICA, health insurance);
- volume and price changes for supplies and drugs;
- purchased services and malpractice costs (professional fees);
- location lease or ownership costs, utilities, and so on;
- cost of borrowing (interest expense); and
- systems development.

The historical cost is a place to start for information, but the group should be aware of changes that are occurring. Recent years have seen malpractice insurance premium increases of 20 percent to 80 percent a year. Health insurance costs are increasing at 10 percent to 20 percent per year. The nursing shortage has made it difficult to hire registered nurses, exerting pressure on salaries and benefits. When cost increases of these proportions occur and the reimbursement side of the profit equation is not increasing as rapidly, other ways to generate revenue must be considered.

Capital Budgeting

Capital Requirements for Medical Groups

The need for capital in medical groups includes financing for equipment, leasehold improvements, and working capital. Smaller medical groups have tended not to perform capital budgeting, and they finance equipment and other capital expenditures by 100-percent loans. Banks and other lenders are willing to lend money to medical groups because of their excellent credit risk. Banks often request and receive personal guarantees from the physician shareholders.

Medium-sized groups tend to begin to build capital internally through the retention of profits, but they must also depend on bank financing.

Larger medical groups (150 or more providers) tend to have higher capital needs because office space needs are greater and they require space specifically built to their needs. They may move toward the bond markets and thus are required to retain capital to meet its covenant requirements.

Examples of ratios that should be evaluated by larger groups are:

$$\text{Operating Margin} = \frac{\text{Income from Operations (Before Investment Income)}}{\text{Patient Service and Other Operating Revenues}}$$

$$\text{Debt Service Coverage} = \frac{\text{Net Income} + \text{Depreciation} + \text{Interest Expense}}{\text{Principal Payments} + \text{Interest Expense}}$$

$$\text{Debt to Total Capitalization} = \frac{\text{Long-term Debt}}{\text{Long-term Debt} + \text{Net Assets}}$$

$$\text{Cushion} = \frac{\text{Unrestricted Cash and Investments}}{\text{Principal Payments} + \text{Interest Expense}}$$

$$\text{Debt Service \% of Revenues} = \frac{\text{Principal Payments} + \text{Interest Expense}}{\text{Operating Revenues}}$$

Financial Performance Targets

Table 5.5 shows a typical range of financial performance targets for the various key indicators. Organizations requiring facility replacement will often target the low end of the desired range.

TABLE 5.5 Potential Financial Performance Targets

Financial Performance Target	*Acceptable Range*	*Investor Grade (Rated)* 2002 S&P A+/A–	2002 S&P BBB+/BBB–	
Profitability				
Operating Margin	1.0% to 3.0%	1.8%	0.6%	
Liquidity and Cash Flow				
Debt Service Coverage	2.0x to 3.3x+	3.3x	2.7x	*
Cushion Ratio	4.0x to 12.0x+	11.8+	7.6x	*
Leverage				
Debt Service % of Revenues	3.3% to 7.0%	3.3%	3.7%	*
Debt to Capitalization	30.0% to 60.0%	34.4%	43.4%	*

* Desired position = desired ratio position relative to the financial performance target.

Financial and Operating Ratios

Performance Measures

The information contained in the basic financial statements can and should be used to provide insight into the financial strength and earnings capacity of the business. This extends beyond net income and requires that relationships between accounts be examined. While an almost unlimited number of such ratios and comparisons are possible, a relatively small number are traditionally the object of most attention. Financial ratios most often computed to analyze the medical group are as follows.

Months Revenue in Accounts Receivable

$$\frac{\text{Accounts Receivable (Balance Sheet)}}{\text{Average Monthly Gross Revenues}} \quad \frac{5{,}409{,}903}{20{,}775{,}206/12} = \frac{5{,}409{,}903}{1{,}731{,}26} = \frac{3.12}{\text{Months}}$$

This ratio measures the number of months' revenues that are uncollected in accounts receivable, providing an idea of how successful the medical group is in collecting its patient receivables.

Gross Collection Ratio

Gross collections measure the percentage of gross charges for which cash payments were received.

$$\frac{\text{Cash Received from Third-party Payers and Customers (Statement of Cash Flows)}}{\text{Gross Fees (Income Statement)}} \quad \frac{\$14{,}718{,}601}{\$20{,}775{,}206} = 70.9\%$$

This ratio measures the percentage of net charges for which cash payments were received. The net collection paid is calculated the same as gross collection ratio, with the exception of reducing gross fees by any contractual discounts.

$$\frac{\text{Cash Received from Third-party Payers and Customers (Statement of Cash Flows)}}{\text{Net Fees (Income Statement)}} \quad \frac{\$6,133,433}{\$6,180,945} = 99.2\%$$

These ratios can be useful in analyzing third-party reimbursement if calculated separately for each payer to help determine the better payers and ensure that each payer is paying as contracted.

The overhead percentage indicator identifies the group's overhead ratio. It is the percentage of total net revenue expended to cover nonphysician expenses. When subtracted from 100 percent, it identifies the proportion of total cash collections available for physician compensation or future income or investments. Overhead can range from 10 percent to 70 percent depending on the specialty. Hospital-based groups (e.g., medical, anesthesia) have lower overhead percentages; surgery groups (e.g., general surgery, orthopedics) are in the middle range; and primary care is at the higher end.

$$\frac{\text{Total Nonphysician Expenses as \% of Total}}{\text{Cash Collections or Net Revenue}} = \frac{\text{Total Nonphysician Expenses}}{\text{Total Net Revenue}} \times 100$$

Table 5.6 demonstrates detailed accounts receivable aging. It is critical to track aging in medical groups because the probability of collecting fees for services rendered decreases dramatically as the accounts receivable get older. Most third-party payers have language in their contracts that allows them to not pay the provider if the claim is made a certain number of months (three to 12) after the date of service.

Although accounts receivable aging information is not typically found in financial statements, a supplementary aging analysis by payer will measure the ability of the firm to collect payment promptly from third-party payers and customers.

The trending of ratios computed from internal financial data can help an organization spot trends related to its business and market. Other ratios that should be tracked for physician groups include RVUs produced. A wealth of information can then be computed and trended

- RVUs produced by full-time equivalent (FTE) physician or provider
- Charges per RVU
- Receipts per RVU
- Total overhead expense per RVU

TABLE 5.6
Accounts
Receivable
Aging by Payer
Type

	Current	31–60 Days	61–90 Days	91–120 Days	120+ Days	Total
Patient	$ 51,903	$ 2,244	$ 12,358	$ 6,179	$ 30,895	$ 123,577
Commercial	46,712	20,019	11,122	5,561	27,805	111,219
BlueCross/ BlueShield	35,034	15,015	8,341	4,171	20,854	83,414
HMO/PPO:						
Blue Plus	108,995	46,712	25,951	12,976	64,878	259,511
Preferred One	10,380	4,449	2,472	1,236	6,179	24,715
Group Health	7,785	3,336	1,854	927	4,634	18,536
Med Centers	6,488	2,780	1,545	772	3,862	15,447
Medica Choice	54,497	23,356	12,976	6,488	32,439	129,755
Medica Primary	44,117	18,907	10,504	5,252	26,260	105,040
Ethix Midwest	3,893	1,668	927	463	2,317	9,268
Select Care	2,595	1,112	618	309	1,545	6,179
Medicare	86,936	37,258	20,699	10,350	51,748	206,991
Medical Assistance	6,488	2,780	1,545	772	3,862	15,447
Workers' Compensation	43,200	22,800	12,667	6,333	31,667	126,666
Total	$519,022	$222,438	$123,577	$61,788	$308,942	$1,235,766
% of Total Receivables		42%	8%	10%	5%	25%

Tools Available

In order to properly analyze the above financial information and ratios it is necessary to compare the group's information to that of similar organizations. Various studies are available for this purpose:

- MGMA Cost Survey
- MGMA Physician Compensation and Production Survey
- MGMA Academic Practice Faculty Compensation and Production Survey
- AMGA Group Practice Compensation Trends and Productivity Correlations
- AMA Socioeconomic Characteristics of a Medical Practice

Potential Uses for Statistical Information

Many groups create management reports and compare their operating results to themselves and to survey data. The surveys track a lot information and provide benchmarks in the areas shown in Figure 5.6.

FIGURE 5.6

Benchmark
Data Provided
by Surveys

Comparison of Operating Cost Data	Comparison of Physician Compensation
Per FTE Physician	By Specialty
As a Percentage of Net Revenue (by Capitation Contract Revenue Percentage)	Starting Salary
	By Years in Specialty
Multi- or Single-specialty Group (Large, Small, Better Performing)	By Group Type (Single- or Multispecialty)
By Geographic Region	By Size of Group
By Legal Organization (Partnership, Professional Organization, Not-for profit)	By Geographic Section
	By Gender
	By Method of Compensation (Salary or Production Based)
	By Percentage of Revenue from At-risk Managed Care Revenue

Comparison of Midlevel Provider Compensation
(Nurse Practitioner, Therapist, Social Worker)
   Similar Data as for Physicians

Comparison of Physician Production
   Same as Physician Compensation
   Resource-based Relative Value Units (RBRVUs)

Comparison of Midlevel Provider Production
(Nurse Practitioner, Therapist, Social Worker)
   Similar Data as for Physicians

Comparison of Accounts Receivable Data, Collection Percentages, and
Financial Ratios

Comparison of Gross Charges by Payer Type

Comparison of Charges and Revenue	Comparison of Staffing, Patients, Charges, and Cost
Per FTE Physician	Nonsurgical Encounters
Per Square Foot	Surgery and Anesthesia Cases
Per RBRVU	Diagnostic Medical and Imaging Procedures
Per Patient	Clinical Laboratory and Pathology Procedures

Taxation and Organization Structure

For income tax reporting, a medical group is considered a professional services corporation if it is independent (owned by physicians).

C corporations are one of the most common types of structure for medical
groups. A C corporation is a traditional tax-paying corporation, as opposed
to a pass-through entity such as an S corporation or partnership. The corporation must pay taxes on taxable income at a federal tax rate of 35 percent.

C Corporations

TABLE 5.7
Corporate and
Professional
Service Tax
Rates

Taxable Income	Tax on Base	Rate*
Corporate Tax Rates		
$0–$50,000	0	15%
$50,000–$75,000	7,500	25%
$75,000–$100,000	13,750	34%
$100,000–$335,000	22,350	39%
More than $18.3 million	6,400,000	35%
Professional Tax Rates		
$0–$50,000	0	35%
$50,000–$75,000	7,500	35%
$75,000–$100,000	13,750	35%
$100,000–$335,000	22,350	25%
More than $18.3 million	6,400,000	35%

*Plus this percentage multiplied by the amount over the bracket base level.

Unlike other business corporations it pays 35 percent on the first dollar earned. The tax tables in Table 5.7 demonstrate the differences between professional service businesses, such as a medical practice, and other industries.

Professional Service Corporations

Professional service corporations do not have the benefit of graduated tax rates. Congress removed this benefit because of concerns that smaller medical groups and incorporated solo practitioners were accumulating profits inside C corporations solely because the corporate rates were lower than the individual rates. Physicians would forgo bonuses and thus corporate profits would be higher; however, the corporate tax was lower than the individual tax.

S Corporations

S corporations are known as pass-through entities because they do not pay corporate income taxes; however, the individual shareholders must pay taxes on the profits at the individual level (i.e., the profits are passed through the corporation to the individual). The benefits of being an S corporation are great if an organization has high level of profits or sells its assets. S corporations are limited in the number of shareholders they can have.

LLCs and LLPs

Limited Liability Corporations (LLCs) and Limited Liability Partnerships (LLPs) are known as hybrid organization because they have the characteristics of a corporation (limited liability) and a partnership (pass-through taxation).

Not-for-profit Organizations

Not-for-profit organizations are exempt from income taxes under the IRS code. Many large medical groups are structured as not-for-profits in order to retain profits without paying taxes and secure tax-exempt bonds at lower interest rates.

If an organization is not-for-profit, it must have outside board members, with few exceptions, and must fulfill certain charitable, research, and educational purposes. There are no owners of a not-for-profit medical group; it is owned by the community, and if the organization ceases to exist and liquidates, its assets must go to another not-for-profit organization.

The compensation of the physicians must be overseen by the outside board members to protect against private inurement. Private inurement regulations prevent insiders of an exempt organization (e.g., members, officers, directors, trustees) from capitalizing on their positions for personal gain. Because of the potential for abuse by insiders, inurement analysis is strict; any inurement of net earnings to an insider, however slight, subjects the organization to revocation of its tax-exempt status or significant sanctions.

Medical Group Valuations

Buy-in and Buy-out Transactions Between Physicians

Common methods for the valuation of the stock related to professional entities are the easy-in/easy-out, book value, and adjusted book value methods. There may be a goodwill component to the buy-in, most often in groups with high income levels. Goodwill has become less common in recent years because group sizes have grown and the need to recruit physicians has made it less likely for a physician to be willing to pay goodwill.

Easy-in/ Easy-out

The easy-in/easy-out method is simply a fixed amount to buy into the corporation, and the buy-out is the same. This can be $1,000 or $50,000. The advantages to this approach are that it is simple and there is no cost to calculate the buy-in and buy-out. In addition such a model can serve as a recruitment incentive if the buy-in price is low enough. Groups that use this method believe that the physician earns her income during her career and that no individual should profit from the buy-in of a colleague.

The disadvantage to the easy-in/easy-out method is that there is no incentive for a physician to invest in the practice as she nears retirement. To invest in equipment or a new location merely reduces the individual physician's compensation, and there is no hope to recoup the investment in the form of a buy-out.

Book Value and Adjusted Book Value

Table 5.8 shows the calculation associated with the book value and adjusted book value methods. These fairly simple methods require little cost to calculate. They do provide some opportunity to reflect the value of equipment purchases.

The difference between the adjusted book value and book value methods relates to the value of the equipment. These methods are chosen

TABLE 5.8

Adjusted Book
Value Example

Radiology Consultants, PA
Buy-in/Buy-out Calculation

Assets

Cash	$650,000
Miscellaneous Receivables	78,000
Prepaid Insurance	122,000
Furniture, Fixture, Equipment	100,000
Leasehold Improvements	200,000
Less Accumulated Depreciation	(275,000)
Net Furniture, Fixture, and Equipment and Leasehold Improvements	25,000
Total Assets	$875,000

Liabilities

Accrued Retirement Plan	$625,000
Accrued Payroll	40,000
Major Accounts Payable	0
Total Liabilities	665,000
Net Assets	210,000
Add-back Half of Accumulated Depreciation	137,500
Adjusted Book Value	347,500
Divided by No. of Shareholders	7
(6 + 1 Buying in)	
Per Shareholder Value if Cross-purchase	$ 49,643
Per Shareholder Value if New Shares	$ 57,917

NOTES:

1. Patient accounts receivable (A/R) are not included in this calculation. Some groups are finding it difficult to charge new physicians for A/R and have stopped doing so in order to make recruitment easier. Other groups handle the A/R buy-in through a separate calculation and manage it through compensation reduction as discussed later in the chapter.

2. Note that the buy-in price is different if the payment goes to the practice for new shares versus going to the existing shareholders (a cross-purchase). The buy-in is greater because the new shareholder will own part of the cash being contributed. If the practice were to distribute the cash, the new shareholder would share in it and thus should pay more. If the buy-in is structured as a cross-purchase, the practice does not increase in value, resulting in a lower price. It is highly recommended that the payments on a buy-in go to the practice as opposed to the existing shareholders. This serves as long-term capital for the practice and helps fund buy-outs as physicians retire. If the payout goes to individual physicians, they should individually buy out other physicians as they retire (which is difficult to do).

when the group believes that the value of the equipment is greater than that shown on the tax return or financial statements (because of rapid deprecation methods) and therefore adjusts these values to be a better approximation of fair-market value. The adjusted book value method states that a piece of equipment will never be valued below 50 percent of cost if it is still being used. This is a simple method, but it may result in overvaluation of the equipment.

Another method is to keep separate depreciation schedules that choose longer lives for some of the equipment. Using a ten-year straight line with a 20-percent residual value is a method that has gained acceptance for many groups. High-tech assets could use a shorter life.

These methods may become complex as a practice grows and adds large amounts of equipment and leasehold improvements. It is important to emphasize that all methods are approximations of the value and should not be treated as a science. Rounding the value to the nearest thousand can help reinforce this concept.

Accounts Receivable or Deferred Compensation

The second component of the buy-in for a medical practice often relates to the accounts receivable buy-in. A major difference compared to a stock buy-in is that the accounts receivable buy-in is commonly done with pretax dollars. The buy-in payments are shifted through salary reductions to the original shareholders. It is important an attorney with a good understanding of the tax issues associated with these transactions draft these and any legal agreements. Documents must be drafted in accordance with appropriate revenue sources, codes, and regulations to ensure that they are treated properly.

The common methods related to accounts receivable or deferred compensation are:

- No buy-in/no buy-out
- Vesting
- Traditional buy-in
- Frozen accounts receivable method

No Buy-in/ No Buy-out

The no buy-in/no buy-out method has been used as a negotiated arrangement when groups are having difficulty recruiting physicians. It also tends to be seen in larger groups. The advantages are that it is simple and promotes recruitment. The disadvantage is that often a fairness issue arises if some of the original physicians bought into the accounts receivable or incurred the cost of the ramping up of accounts receivable when the practice started. If there is no buy-in, usually there is no buy-out or deferred compensation payment when a physician leaves the practice.

Vesting

The vesting method is similar to the no buy-in method; however, when a physician leaves the group, he shares in the accounts receivable. To protect itself the group uses a vesting schedule. The vesting schedules range from 10 percent per year for ten years to 0 percent over the first five years and then 20 percent per year. If a physician leaves the practice during the vesting period, he would receive a prorated share of the accounts receivable multiplied by their vested percentage.

This fairly straightforward method aids in the recruitment of physicians. The disadvantage is that the buy-in does not match the buy-out. The individual physician buying in did not pay for the accounts receivable, yet he receives them when he retires or leaves the practice.

Frozen Accounts Receivable

This method involves no buy-in to the accounts receivable, but the physician buys in shares in the increase of the accounts receivable as of the effective date she became a shareholder. For example, assume the accounts receivable are worth $1 million on the effective date of the buy-in, and this is the tenth physician to be an active shareholder in the group. If the accounts receivable went to $1.2 million, and the most recent physician to become a shareholder left the organization, she would share in one-tenth of the $200,000 increase. A physician who had been a shareholder the entire time and left the organization would receive $131,111 (one-ninth of 1 million plus one-tenth of $200,000).

This method can become quite complex as the number of shareholders increases and multiple layers are created over many years. In addition accounts receivable may decrease over time; thus when an individual leaves the practice, in theory she could owe the other partners money related to accounts receivable valuation.

Income Distribution Formulas

Many groups have moved away from exact computations related to accounts receivable buy-ins. Instead, after one to two years the associate goes from straight salary to receiving compensation equal to a percentage of a full shareholder's compensation level for several years. Some examples include:

- 60 percent the first year, 80 percent the second year, and 100 percent the third year; or
- 80 percent the first year, 90 percent the second year, 95 percent the third year, and 100 percent the fourth year.

The deferred compensation payout tends to be a percentage of the final W-2. This approach is straightforward, and it reduces the complexities and potential disagreements related to the purchase of accounts receivable. Depending on the percentages used, the amount can be approximately equal to a prorated share of the accounts receivable or potentially greater.

Valuation of Ancillary Entities

Medical groups have expanded into new areas such as imaging centers, ambulatory surgery centers, optical eyewear sales, hearing aid dispensaries, and other business lines. Some groups view these business lines as different from the professional practice and choose a different valuation method. These activities are different because the profits are not dependent on physician services, but rather relate to the investment of capital and fees charged for technical equipment or the market on retail sales.

If an organization does choose to value the business lines differently, an earnings multiple is used to estimate the value of buy-ins and buy-outs. A general guideline for earnings multiples is three to seven times earnings before interest expense, depreciation, taxes, and amortization. Many practices choose to be on the low side for valuations of their buy/sell agreements to make it more affordable for physicians to join the group.

Retirement Benefits for Physicians

The retirement benefit is sometimes called the sacred cow of medical groups. MGMA compensation surveys show that physician retirement benefits average $28,000 to $40,000 per year. The ability to defer taxes is extremely important to physicians. If an organization cuts back on this benefit, there will most certainly be trouble. Deferred income provides security for the physician in the long run.

Retirement plans can be qualified or nonqualified. The IRS and Department of Labor approve qualified plans. A plan will be approved if it provides benefits to all eligible employees and does not discriminate in favor of highly compensated employees or officers of the organization. The benefit of a qualified plan is that the organization receives a tax deduction for the funds placed in the retirement accounts, and the individual does not pay tax on the money until it is withdrawn. Another advantage is that the funds are deductible as an expense to the corporation.

An advantage for not-for-profit organizations is that they can add nonqualified retirement plans without losing the tax deduction.

Qualified Retirement Plans

There are three main types of qualified retirement plans:

- defined contribution;
- defined benefit; and
- hybrid.

Defined Contribution

A defined contribution plan is the most common type of retirement plan in medical groups. Contribution is calculated and contributed to each individual's account. The future retirement benefit is determined by the investment results of the individual account.

The most common defined contribution plans include 401(k), profit-sharing, and pension plans.

401(k) plans

401(k) plans allow individuals to reduce their individual compensation by up to $14,000 and contribute it to a retirement account. The contribution (deferred income) is not subject to individual income tax until the funds are withdrawn at retirement. Many organizations match some portion of the 401(k). For example, the organization will match 50 percent of the first 6

TABLE 5.9
Employer-
matched
401(k) Plan

Compensation	Employee Deferral at 6%	Employer Match at 50%	Total
$30,000	$ 1,800	$ 900	$ 2,700
$40,000	$ 2,400	$1,200	$ 3,600
$50,000	$ 3,000	$1,500	$ 4,500
$75,000	$ 4,500	$2,250	$ 6,750
$100,000	$ 6,000	$3,000	$ 9,000
$150,000	$ 9,000	$4,500	$13,500
$200,000	$12,000	$6,000	$18,000
$210,000	$12,600	$6,300	$18,900

percent of compensation that an employee contributes, as shown in Table 5.9. The match creates an incentive for individuals to contribute to their own retirement.

Profit-sharing plans   A profit-sharing plan is often provided in conjunction with a 401(k) plan. An organization can contribute additional funds to the retirement account at its discretion. The contribution is then allocated among the eligible employees. Sometimes the contribution is calculated based on a percentage of employee wages (between 0 and 25 percent of wages). Defined contribution plan contributions cannot exceed $40,000 for an individual. The maximum compensation used for computation purposes was $210,000 for 2004. The IRS adjusts this rate annually.

Many for-profit groups go through a process of calculating the maximum for highly compensated individuals. A simple computation is shown in Table 5.10.

It is apparent that the benefit becomes quite rich. It is rare for organizations to contribute more than 10 percent to profit sharing, as employees who make more than $210,000 would not receive any of the funds because they would be above the maximum individual contribution of $40,000.

Pension plan   A defined contribution pension plan is similar to a profit-sharing plan, with the major difference being that the amount of the contribution is fixed as a percentage of wages. For example, 5 percent of wages will be contributed each year. A pension plan does not have the flexibility of a profit-sharing plan's discretionary contributions.

Defined Benefit   A defined benefit plan is a retirement plan that defines how much an individual will receive per month after retirement. The organization must contribute sufficient funds to achieve this goal. The benefit (e.g., $3,000 per month) as opposed to the contribution is defined. The benefit is determined most often based on a combination of three factors: age, length of service, and compensation. Actuaries calculate the funding requirements, taking into account expected investment returns and life expectancies.

The hybrid plans combine some of the features of a defined contribution and defined benefit plan. Some common hybrid plans are known as target benefit plans and cash balance plans.

Hybrid

Compliance Requirements

The federal Employee Retirement Income Security Act (ERISA) of 1974 sets requirements for retirement and health plans to provide protection for individuals enrolled in them. ERISA requires plans to provide participants with plan information about their investments and options. Plans with more than 100 participants are required to be audited by an independent accounting firm. The administration of retirement plans has become more complex over the years, and there are professionals who specialize in the legal, accounting, and investment areas.

Summary

This chapter provides the information necessary to understand the unique differences in financial management of group practices. The revenue streams from reimbursement are highly regulated, and costs are difficult to contain. The American public has an insatiable appetite for a finite resource. The importance of a fundamental understanding of accounting is demonstrated throughout the discussions. The characteristics of the financial statements provide insights into the similarities as well as the differences between group practice and other healthcare and business organizations. Both capital and operating statements are covered, as are the myriad regulations that govern

Compensation	Employee Deferral at 6%	Employer Match at 50%	Profit Sharing at 10%	Total
$ 30,000	$ 1,800	$ 900	$ 3,000	$ 5,700
$ 40,000	$ 2,400	$1,200	$ 4,000	$ 7,600
$ 50,000	$ 3,000	$1,500	$ 5,000	$ 9,500
$ 75,000	$ 4,500	$2,250	$ 7,500	$14,250
$100,000	$ 6,000	$3,000	$10,000	$19,000
$150,000	$ 9,000	$4,500	$15,000	$28,500
$200,000	$12,000	$6,000	$20,000	$38,000
$210,000	$12,600	$6,300	$21,000	$39,900

TABLE 5.10
Computation of Maximums for a Defined Contribution Plan

group practice financial systems, especially on the reimbursement side. A key to understanding the ratios important to group practices is also provided along with the special consideration related to compliance.

Discussion Questions

1. What makes accounting for physician groups unique?
2. What are some of the problems with the current methods for reimbursement for medical services?
3. Why are valuation methods important for physician groups?
4. What are the criteria to become a 501(c)(3) organization?
5. Describe the difference between a professional corporation and a partnership from the tax perspective.
6. Describe the difference between a deferred contribution and defined benefit retirement plan.

References

American Medical Association. 2002. *Current Procedural Terminology (CPT®)*. Chicago: AMA Press.

Coddington, D. C. 2001. "Integrated Healthcare Is Alive and Well." *Frontiers of Health Services Management* 17 (4): 31–40.

Hsiao, W. C., P. Braun, D. L. Dunn, E. R. Becker, et al. 1992. "An Overview of the Development and Refinement of the RBRVS—The Foundation for Reform of U.S. Physician Payment." *Medical Care Supplement* 30 (11): NS1–12.

Piland, N., and K. P. Glass (Eds.). 1999. *Chart of Accounts for Health Care Organizations*. Englewood, CO: Medical Group Management Association.

APPENDIX 5.1 SAMPLE FINANCIAL REPORTS

Board of Directors and Stockholders
Minnesota Medical, PA
Home Town, Minnesota

We have reviewed the accompanying balance sheets of Minnesota Medical, PA, as of December 31, 2002 and 2001, and the related statements of income and retained earnings, and cash flows for the years then ended, in accordance with Statements on Standards for Accounting and Review Services issued by the American Institute of Certified Public Accountants. All information included in these financial statements is the representation of the management of Minnesota Medical, PA.

A review consists principally of inquiries of company personnel and analytical procedures applied to financial data. It is substantially less in scope than an audit in accordance with generally accepted auditing standards, the objective of which is the expression of an opinion regarding the financial statements taken as a whole. Accordingly, we do not express such an opinion.

Based on our reviews, with the exception of the matter described in the following paragraph, we are not aware of any material modifications that should be made to the accompanying financial statements in order for them to be in conformity with generally accepted accounting principles.

Our review was made for the purpose of expressing limited assurance that there are no material modifications that should be made to the financial statements in order for them to be in conformity with generally accepted accounting principles. The information included on pages 10 through 13 is presented only for supplementary analysis purposes. Such information has been subjected to the inquiry and analytical procedures applied in the review of the basic financial statements, and we are not aware of any material modifications that should be made thereto. The information on page 14 is presented only for supplementary analysis purposes and has not been subjected to the inquiry and analytical procedures applied in the review of the basic financial statements, but was compiled from information that is the representation of management, without audit or review. Accordingly, we do not express an opinion or any other form of assurance on it.

Minneapolis, Minnesota
February 13, 2003

LARSON, ALLEN, WEISHAIR & CO., LLP

Minnesota Medical, PA: Balance Sheets December 31, 2002 and 2001
(See Accountant's Review Report)

Assets	2002	2001
Current Assets		
Cash	$ 428,466	$ 435,700
Accounts Receivable—Net	2,508,552	2,037,070
Reserve Receivables from Third-Party Payers	299,326	531,521
Notes Receivable		−10,431
Taxes Receivable		−23,918
Prepaid Insurance		−66,684
Inventory	50,000	50,000
Total Current Assets	$3,286,344	$ 3,155,324
Property and Equipment		
Leasehold Improvements	$ 223,203	$ 219,576
Furniture and Equipment	1,388,684	1,191,809
Total Property and Equipment	$ 1,611,887	$ 1,411,385
Less: Accumulated Depreciation	1,169,370	993,703
Net Property and Equipment	$ 442,517	$ 417,682
Other Assets		
Other Assets	$ 31,517	$ 16,000
Total Assets	$3,760,378	$ 3,589,006
Current Liabilities		
Accounts Payable	$ 174,704	$ 117,674
Patient Refunds Payable	256,956	200,000
Current Portion of Long-Term Debt	92,640	106,791
Deferred Compensation Plan	780,000	784,000
Accrued Salaries and Vacation	446,530	406,776
Accrued Retirement Plan	473,562	693,982
Accrued MN Care Taxes	2,000	65,277
Other Current Liabilities	43,218	20,749
Total Current Liabilities	$ 2,269,610	$ 2,395,249
Long-Term Liabilities		
Long-Term Debt (Net of Current Maturities)	$ 371,780	—
Total Long-Term Liabilities	$ 371,780	—
Total Liabilities	$ 2,641,390	$ 2,395,249
Stockholder's Equity		
Common Stock, $10 Par Value; 23,000 and 25,000		
Shares Issued and Outstanding, Respectively	$ 230,000	$ 250,000
Retained Earnings	888,988	943,757
Total Stockholder's Equity	$ 1,118,988	$ 1,193,757
Total Liabilties and Stockholder's Equity	$ 3,70,378	$ 3,589,006

See accompanying Notes to Financial Statements

Minnesota Medical, PA: Statement of Income and Retained Earnings
for the Years Ended December 31, 2002 and 2001
(See Accountant's Review Report)

	2002		2001	
	Amount	*% of Net Revenues*	*Amount*	*% of Net Revenues*
Net Revenues	$ 14,635,661	100.00%	$14,686,176	100.00%
Operating Expenses				
Human Resources	$ 5,489,875	37.70%	$ 5,043,506	34.20%
Physical Resources	2,597,328	17.70%	2,442,146	16.60%
Purchased Services	726,850	5.00%	506,904	3.60%
General and Administrative	598,081	4.20%	555,744	3.80%
Total Operating Expenses	$ 9,412,134	64.60%	$ 8,548,300	58.20%
Operating Income	$ 5,223,527	35.40%	$ 6,137,876	41.80%
Physician's Salaries and Benefits	(5,370,376)	36.80%	(6,114,904)	41.60%
Income (Loss) Before Other Income	$ (146,849)	(1.40)%	$ 22,972	0.20%
Other Income	92,080	0.60%	141,454	0.90%
Net Income (Loss)	$ (54,769)	(0.80)%	$ 164,426	1.10%
Retained Earnings—Beginning	943,757		779,331	
Retained Earnings	$ 888,988		$ 943,757	

See accompanying Notes to Financial Statements

**Minnesota Medical, PA: Statements of Cash Flows
for the Years Ended December 31, 2002 and 2001
(See Accountant's Review Report)**

	2002	2001
Cash Flows from Operating Activities		
Net Income (Loss)	$ (54,769)	$ 164,426
Adjustments to Reconcile Net Loss to Net		
Cash Provided by Operating Activities:		
Depreciation	175,667	148,912
Net (Increase) Decrease in Current Assets:		
Accounts Receivable	(471,482)	175,763
Notes Receivable	10,431	(6,431)
Reserve Receivables from Third-Party Payers	232,195	(531,521)
Taxes Receivable	23,918	(23,918)
Prepaid Insurance	66,684	(7,395)
Other Assets	(14,517)	—
Net Increase (Decrease) in Current Liabilities:		
Accounts Payable	57,030	(71,469)
Patient Refunds	56,957	25,000
Deferred Compensation Payable	(4,000)	98,000
Accrued Salaries and Vacation	39,754	28,744
Accrued Pension and Profit Sharing	(282,361)	600,095
Accrued MN Care Taxes	(63,277)	5,277
Income Taxes payable	—	(41,500)
Other Current Liabilities	84,410	(446)
Net Cash Provided (Used) by Operating Activities	$ (143,360)	$ 563,537
Cash Flows from Investing Activities		
Investment in Partnership	$ (1,000)	$ (12,000)
Acquisition of Equipment	(200,502)	(113,415)
Net Cash Used by Investing Activities	$ (201,502)	$ (125,415)
Cash Flows from Financing Activities		
Advance Received from Line of Credit	$ 300,000	—
Payments Received from Notes Payable	500,000	—
Payments on Line of Credit	(300,000)	—
Payments on Notes Payable	(162,372)	(129,060)
Net Cash Provided (Used) by Financing Activities	337,628	(129,060)
Net Increase (Decrease) in Cash and Cash Equivalents	$ (2,234)	$ 309,062
Cash and Cash Equivalents—Beginning	435,700	126,638
Cash and Cash Equivalents—Ending	$ 428,466	$ 435,700

See accompanying Notes to Financial Statements

Minnesota Medical, PA: Notes to Financial Statements
December 31, 2002 and 2001
(See Accountant's Review Report)

Note 1: Summary of Significant Accounting Policies

Nature of Business
Minnesota Medical, PA, owns and operates a multispecialty clinic in Minnesota.

Basis of Financial Statement Presentation
The Corporation prepares its financial statements on the accrual basis of accounting, except for deferred income taxes and salaries as described in Note 8, which is a generally accepted accounting principle.

Cash and Cash Equivalent
For purposes of the financial statements, the Corporation considers all short-term debt securities purchased with original maturities of three months or less to be cash equivalents.

Accounts Receivable
Accounts receivable are accounted for using the allowance method. An allowance is provided for both doubtful accounts and contractual and statutory discounts and adjustments.

Depreciation
The cost of property and equipment is depreciated using accelerated methods over estimated useful lives of five to seven years for furniture, fixtures, and computer equipment.

Use of Estimates
The preparation of financial statements in conformity with generally accepted accounting principles requires management to make estimates and assumptions that affect the reported amounts of assets and liabilities and disclosure of contingent assets and liabilities at the date of the financial statements. Estimates also affect the reported amounts of revenue and expense during the reporting period. Actual results could differ from those estimates.

Concentration of Credit Risk
The Corporation maintains cash accounts with a high-credit-quality financial institution. At times cash balances may be in excess of the FDIC insurance limits.
   The Corporation performs periodic evaluations of its clients' financial condition and generally does not require collateral. Substantially all receivables are due from third-party payers and patients.

Note 2: Accounts Receivable

	2002	2001
Accounts Receivable	$ 5,409,903	$ 3,799,405
Less: Allowance for Doubtful Accounts, Contractual and Statutory Discounts, and Adjustments	(2,901,351)	(1,72,335)
Total	$ 2,508,552	$ 2,307,070

Notes 3: Notes Payable

Description	2002	2001
Note Payable—First Bank; Monthly Principle and Interest Payments of $10,440; Interest Rate of 9.25%; Due April 2007; Secured by All Equipment and Accounts Receivable	$ 447,190	$ —
Note Payable—Shareholders; Monthly Principle and Interest Payments of $886; Interest Rate of 6%; Due August 2004; Unsecured	$ 17,230	—
Note Payable—First National Bank; Monthly Principal and Interest Payments of $11,073; Interest rate of 7.8%; Due September 2002; Secured by All Equipment and Accounts	—	101,147
Note Payable—Shareholders; Monthly Principal and Interest Payments of $886; Interest Rate of 6%; Due September 2002	—	5,644
Total	$ 464,420	$ 106,791
Less: Current Portion	(92,640)	(106,791)
Long-Term Portion	$ 371,780	$ —

Future annual principal maturities on the above notes payable are as follows:

Year Ending December 31	Amount
2003	$ 92,640
2004	99,623
2005	105,438
2006	115,616
2007	51,003
Therafter	—
Total	$ 464,320

Note 4: Line of Credit

The Corporation maintains a $400,000 line of credit with First Bank. The interest rate is variable. The balance due on this line as of December 31, 2002 and 2001 was $–0-.

Note 5: Money Purchase Pension Plan

The Corporation has a money purchase pension plan that covers substantially all employees that meet certain age and length-of-service requirements. The plan provides that an annual contribution based on a formula of qualifying employees' annual compensation (subject to certain limitations) will be contributed to the plan. The required contributions for the years ended December 31, 2002 and 2001 were $416,633 and $518,026, respectively.

Note 6: Profit-Sharing Plan

The Corporation has a profit-sharing plan that covers substantially all employees that meet certain age and length-of-service requirements. The plan provides that the Corporation may make an annual contribution to the plan up to the maximum amount allowable by the IRS code. Contributions to the plan are at the discretion of the Board of Directors. Contributions for the years ended December 31, 2002 and 2001 were $-o- and $108,865, respectively.

The Company has adopted a deferred salary reduction arrangement intended to qualify under IRS code section 401(k). Participating employees may elect to defer up to 10 percent of their salaries. The Company matches 50 percent of the employee's contribution up to 2 percent of compensation. Contributions for the years ended December 31, 2002 and 2001 were $115,687 and $106,346, respectively.

Note 7: Operating Lease

The Corporation leased office space from a related party until July 30, 2002. On July 30, 2002 the related party was purchased by an unrelated party. The new lease agreement expires on May 31, 2016, and the base rent is as follows:

	Annual Rent
August 2001–July 2006	$ 724,500
August 2006–July 2011	724,500
August 2011–July 2016	724,500

Rent expense under the current lease was $287,500 for the year ended December 31, 2002.

Total future minimum rental payments under the above operating lease as of December 31, 2002 were as follows:

Year Ending December 31	*Amount*
2002	$ 690,000
2003	690,000
2004	690,000
2005	690,000
2006	704,375
Total	$ 3,464,375

Note 8: Commitments

Stock Purchase Agreements
Under the terms of an agreement with its stockholders the Corporation is required to purchase their shares upon death, termination, or other defined circumstances. The purchase price paid for the shares shall be $100 per share.

Deferred Compensation Agreements
The Corporation has deferred compensation agreements with shareholders that provide benefits upon their voluntary or involuntary termination. The amount payable to each shareholder is based on years of service and scaled to the maximum of $44,000 for ten or more years of service.

The balances of deferred compensation payable at December 31, 2002 and 2001 were $780,000 and $784,000, respectively.

Note 9: Income Taxes

The provision for income taxes consists of the following:

	2002	*2001*
Current Income Taxes:		
Federal	$ 0	$ 0
State	0	0
Total	$ 0	$ 0

The Corporation does not record deferred income taxes on the temporary differences between financial statement and taxable income as required by generally accepted accounting principles. Temporary differences arise from the recognition of income and expenses when cash is received or paid for income tax purposes and the recognition of income when earned and expenses when incurred for financial reporting purposes. The impact on the financial statements for this departure from generally accepted accounting principles is not known at this time.

Note 10: Contingencies

During 2001 the Corporation started a self-insured health plan for its employees. This plan was terminated beginning in 2002. Estimated future claims for incurred medical services of approximately $32,100 were recorded as a liability at December 31, 2001.

Minnesota Medical, PA: Supplementary Comparative Schedules of Net Revenues, Human Resource Expenses, and Physical Resource Expenses for theYears Ended December 31, 2002 and 2001 (See Accountant's Report on Supplementary Information)

	2002		2001	
	Amount	% of Net Revenues	Amount	% of Net Revenues
Revenues				
Gross Charges	$ 20,775,206	151.9%	$18,386,317	125.1%
Discounts and Allowances	(6,076,970)	(41.5)	(3,936,471)	(26.8)
Reserve Revenue	299,326	2.0	531,521	3.6
Patient Refunds	(95,751)	(0.7)	(65,367)	(0.4)
MN Care Taxes	(266,150)	(1.8)	(229,824)	1.6
Net Revenues	$ 14,635,661	100.0%	$14,686,176	100.0%
Human Resource Expenses				
Salaries	$ 4,618,164	31.6%	$ 4,194,727	28.6%
Payroll Taxes	386,168	2.6	343,488	2.3
Profit-Sharing Contribution	54,081	0.4	76,297	0.5
Pension Contribution	210,950	1.4	227,932	1.5
Auto	7,618	0.1	6,297	—
Education	4,062	—	7,511	0.1
Medical Reimbursement	(146)	—	128	—
Health Insurance	69,265	0.5	63,624	0.4
Life Insurance	32,189	0.2	47,412	0.3
Disability Insurance	67,285	0.5	28,206	0.2
Worker's Comp Insurance	9,767	0.1	11,245	0.1
Other Employee Benefits	23,049	0.2	20,579	0.1
Dues and Subscriptions	7,423	0.1	16,088	0.1
Total Human Resource Expenses	$ 5,489,875	37.7%	$5,043,506	34.2%
Physical Resource Expenses				
Medical Supplies	$ 665,193	4.5%	$ 637,697	4.3%
Laboratory Supplies	298,529	2.0	219,130	1.5
X-Ray Supplies	64,696	0.4	58,560	0.4
Building Rent	806,962	5.5	857,468	5.8
Equipment Rent	17,302	0.1	14,548	0.1
Real Estate Taxes	176,231	1.2	181,523	1.2
General Insurance	22,155	0.2	23,811	0.2
Maintenance—Building	24,366	0.2	23,493	0.2
Maintenance—Other	43,593	0.3	10,828	0.1
Maintenance—Equipment	89,334	0.6	103,912	0.7
Telephone	98,711	0.7	72,242	0.5
Paging	4,809	—	2,876	—
Utilities	109,780	0.8	87,146	0.6
Depreciation	175,667	1.2	148,912	1.0
Total Human Resource Expenses	$ 2,597,328	17.7%	$ 2,442,146	16.6%

**Minnesota Medical, PA: Supplementary Comparative Schedules of Purchased
Services and General and Administrative Expenses
for theYears Ended December 31, 2002 and 2001
(See Accountant's Report on Supplementary Information)**

	2002 Amount	2002 % of Net Revenues	2001 Amount	2001 % of Net Revenues
Purchased Services Expenses				
Legal and Accounting	$ 117,547	0.8%	$ 114,156	0.8%
Professional Fees and Licenses	9,933	0.1	4,121	—
Medical Consultant	30,357	0.2	16,964	0.1
Laboratory	344,357	2.4	257,463	1.8
Dietitian	48	—	48	—
Contract Labor	420	—	8,995	0.1
Maintenance Contract	51,142	0.3	29,107	0.2
Payroll Services	16,688	0.1	12,544	0.1
Dictation	48,106	0.3	39,523	0.3
Provider Services	505	—	503	—
Collection and Billing	54,217	0.4	11,911	0.1
Miscellaneous Professional Services	53,141	0.4	11,569	0.1
Total Purchased Services Expenses	$726,850	5.0%	$506,904	3.6%
General and Administrative Expenses				
Laundry and Uniforms	$ 10,567	0.1%	$ 9,802	0.1%
Printing	170,071	1.2	114,777	0.8
Advertising	6,336	—	4,336	—
Office Expense	89,253	0.6	59,530	0.4
Computer Programming	7,194	—	9,812	0.1
Postage and Freight	37,762	0.3	57,915	0.4
Retirement Plan Fees	10,493	0.1	52,917	0.4
Malpractice Insurance	195,677	1.3	194,593	1.3
Moving Expense	—	—	2,000	—
Dues and Subscriptions	1,204	—	3,944	—
Recruitment	9,578	0.1	9,175	0.1
Practice Development	11,300	0.1	5,654	—
Patient Education	8,997	0.1	—	—
Charitable Contributions	4,487	—	4,135	—
Meals and Entertainment	7,867	0.1	14,935	0.1
Meetings and Conferences	11,282	0.1	12,185	0.1
Miscellaneous	16,013	0.1	16	—
Total General and Administrative Expenses	$ 598,081	4.2%	$555,744	3.8%

Minnesota Medical, PA: Supplementary Comparative Schedules of Purchased Services and General and Administrative Expenses (continued) for theYears Ended December 31, 2002 and 2001 (See Accountant's Report on Supplementary Information)

	2002		2001	
	Amount	% of Net Revenues	Amount	% of Net Revenues
Physician's Salaries and Benefits and Outside Specialists				
Physician Salaries	$3,624,958	24.8%	$4,184,196	28.5%
Deferred Compensation	—	—	98,000	0.7
Payroll Taxes	176,163	1.2	172,912	0.7
Profit-Sharing Contributions	61,606	0.4	139,638	1.0
Pension Contributions	205,683	1.4	290,094	2.0
Medical and Life Insurance	82,564	0.6	134,270	0.9
Disability Insurance	27,996	0.2	—	—
Professional Expenses	62,228	0.4	45,893	0.3
Continuing Education	32,187	0.2	29,742	0.2
Books and Subscriptions	471	—	177	—
Meetings, Travel, and Entertainment	39,889	0.3	38,353	0.2
Auto Expenses	—	—	354	—
Special Stipends	25,490	0.2	30,023	0.2
Outside Specialists:				
Gynecology	70,998	0.5	106,375	0.7
EKG Services	7,940	0.1	3,644	—
Ear Nose Throat	343,546	2.3	278,792	1.9
Gastroenterology	128,111	0.9	132,315	0.9
Audiology	52,334	0.4	49,933	0.3
Orthopedics	205,544	1.4	255,821	1.5
Rheumatology	2,038	—	33	—
Allergist	86,625	0.6	57,435	0.4
Radiology	98,188	0.7	96,904	0.7
Surgery	35,817	0.2	—	—
Total Physician Salaries and Benefits and Outside Specialists	$5,370,376	36.8%	$6,114,904	41.6%
Other (Income) Expenses				
Interest Expense	$ 42,027	0.3%	$ 19,459	0.1%
Interest Income	(21,276)	(0.1)	(19,322)	(0.1)
Rental Income	(91,226)	(0.6)	(89,443)	(0.6)
Miscellaneous Income	(25,003)	(0.2)	(62,616)	(0.4)
Penalties	2,538	0.0	0	0.0
Excise Taxes	0	0.0	10,140	0.1
Sales Tax	860	0.0	328	0.0
Total Other (Income) Expenses	$ (92,080)	(0.6)%	$ (141,454)	(0.9)%

APPENDIX 5.2 SAMPLE MANAGEMENT REPORTS

	Year to Date 2004 Budget	Budget % of YTD Income	Year to Date 2004 Actual	Actual % of YTD Income	Year to Date 2003 Actual	Prior Year % of YTD Income
Revenue						
03500.0 • Services Rendered	4,567,030.98		4,782,032.08		4,706,495.16	
03510.0 • Less Discounts	(1,303,343.52)		(1,386,600.45)		(1,318,446.06)	
03520.0 • Less Write Offs and Adjustments	16,678.02		(16,531.69)		5,151.29	
03530.0 • Less Refunds	(16,118.52)		(17,777.41)		(12,465.38)	
03535.0 • Less Refunds	0.00		0.00		(4,860.68)	
03980.0 • Other	0.00		593.36		0.00	
03550.0 • Cash Receipts Reconcilled to A/R	0.00		62,840.18		(52,892.57)	
Total Revenue Collected	3,264,246.96	100.0%	3,424,556.07	100.0%	3,322,981.76	100.0%
Expense						
05000.0 • Human Resources	942,119.80	28.86%	923,358.66	26.96%	910,393.38	27.4%
06100.0 • Physical Resources Expense	151,511.58	4.64%	163,553.75	4.78%	135,787.38	4.09%
06400.0 • Occupancy and Use Expenses	355,840.56	10.9%	349,258.82	10.2%	350,003.65	10.53%
07000.0 • Purchased Services	217,537.02	6.66%	279,484.11	8.16%	228,980.02	6.89%
07400.0 • General and Administrative Exp.	205,083.02	6.28%	97,958.42	2.86%	186,714.25	5.62%
Total Operating Expense	1,872,091.98	57.35%	1,813,613.76	52.96%	1,811,878.68	54.53%

	Year to Date 2004 Budget	Budget % of YTD Income	Year to Date 2004 Actual	Actual % of YTD Income	Year to Date 2003 Actual	Prior Year % of YTD Income
Operating Income	1,392,154.98	42.65%	1,610,942.31	47.04%	1,511,103.08	45.47%
Other Income and (Expense)						
08100.0 • Other Income and Expense	(69,810.48)	(2.14%)	(73,726.35)	(2.15%)	(59,330.62)	(1.79%)
Total Other Income (Expense)	(69,810.48)	(2.14%)	(73,726.35)	(2.15%)	(59,330.62)	(1.79%)
Net Income Before Provider Expenses	1,322,344.50	40.51%	1,537,215.96	44.89%	1,451,772.46	43.69%
Provider Costs						
05050.0 • Nurse Practitioner Expenses	112,013.55	3.43%	117,411.05	3.43%	119,997.25	3.61%
05050.0 • Non-owner M.D. Salaries, Benefits, and Tax	192,230.39	5.89%	119,135.62	3.48%	105,579.80	3.18%
05050.0 • Deferred Compensation Expenses	0.00	0.0%	0.00	0.0%	23,919.05	0.72%
05050.0 • Physicians Salaries, Benefits, and Expenses	1,019,309.51	31.23%	1,046,013.20	30.54%	1,036,234.58	31.18%
Total Provider Costs	1,323,553.45	40.55%	1,282,559.87	37.45%	1,285,730.68	38.69%
Net Income	(1,208.95)	(0.04%)	254,656.09	7.44%	166,041.78	5.0%

MINNESOTA MEDICAL, PA
Summary of Financial Results
August 2004

	Current Year		Prior Year		YTD % Change from Prior			% Change
	Month	YTD	Month	YTD	Year	Goal		from Goal
Gross Charges	2,466,320	16,397,370	2,374,019	15,360,941	6.32	18,000,000		−9.77
Net Receipts	1,050,619	7,718,389	1,144,029	6,858,650	11.14	9,600,000		−24.38
Gross Collection	42.60%	47.07%	48.19%	44.65%	2.42	50.00%		N/A
Net Revenue (Cash to Bank)	965,028	7,161,492	1,047,016	6,129,422	14.41	9,000,000		−25.67
Operating and Administrative	184,985	1,660,139	189,835	1,241,567	25.21	1,800,000		−8.42
Physician Expenses	335,299	4,599,288	294,664	4,119,113	10.44	7,200,000		−56.55
Net Income	444,744	902,066	562,517	768,743	14.78	—		
Average Revenue Per Physician FTE	129,806	863,019	158,268	1,024,063	−15.73			
Average Revenue Per Nonphysician FTE	35,021	257,280	32,687	195,961	23.83			
A/R days	72	72	51	51	29.16			

MINNESOTA MEDICAL, PA
Accounts Receivable Summary

Date	Beginning A/R	Charges	Payments	Adjustments	Ending A/R	Collection (%)	DSO
2002							
Jan	421,519	304,599	179,232	108,323	438,562	58.8	47.6
Feb	438,562	272,360	163,316	84,773	462,833	60.0	51.7
Mar	462,833	262,592	186,403	107,860	431,162	71.0	47.1
Apr	431,162	315,160	211,728	108,664	425,929	67.2	45.9
May	425,929	278,619	202,604	116,154	385,790	72.7	41.0
Jun	385,790	292,297	191,495	90,908	395,684	65.5	41.3
Jul	395,684	294,757	207,610	112,437	370,395	70.4	38.9
Aug	370,395	306,511	190,938	96,560	389,408	62.3	40.1
Sep	389,408	316,337	178,653	94,283	432,809	56.5	43.2
Oct	432,809	305,874	202,927	109,567	426,189	66.3	42.8
Nov	426,189	277,903	184,196	91,655	428,241	66.3	43.0
Dec	428,241	291,531	186,898	121,261	411,613	64.1	41.3
YTD	421,519	3,518,539	2,285,999	1,242,446	411,613	65.0	
2003							
Jan	411,613	355,184	193,089	116,068	457,640	54.4	44.4
Feb	457,640	278,797	163,302	113,786	459,349	58.6	45.3
Mar	459,349	299,719	195,309	106,887	456,464	65.2	45.4
Apr	456,464	313,291	205,345	114,194	450,216	65.5	44.6
May	450,216	293,525	201,195	134,673	407,873	68.5	40.1
Jun	407,873	323,152	179,857	99,323	451,846	55.7	43.6
Jul	451,846	298,045	235,947	135,415	378,529	79.2	37.7
Aug	378,529	320,693	216,903	129,743	352,576	67.6	34.3
Sep	352,576	335,802	189,440	106,983	391,956	56.4	37.4
Oct	391,953	333,423	213,192	122,851	389,333	63.9	36.8
Nov	389,333	282,727	173,893	100,131	398,036	61.5	37.8
Dec	398,036	352,919	197,031	118,507	435,417	55.8	40.7
YTD	411,613	3,787,278	2,364,502	1,398,561	435,827	62.4	

MINNESOTA MEDICAL, PA
Accounts Receivable Summary (continued)

Date	Beginning A/R	Charges	Payments	Adjustments	EndingA/R	Collection (%)	DSO
2004							
Jan	419,471	293,269	184,710	109,523	418,507	63.0	39.3
Feb	418,508	301,707	152,073	91,266	476,876	50.4	45.2
Mar	476,876	353,355	237,372	139,955	452,904	67.2	42.5
Apr	452,904	308,843	218,984	135,062	407,701	70.9	38.8
May	407,701	285,004	196,049	111,196	385,460	68.8	36.6
Jun	385,460	339,714	225,237	120,699	379,238	66.3	36.3
Jul	379,238	328,240	179,899	98,839	428,740	54.8	40.3
Aug					0		0.0
Sep					0		0.0
Oct					0		0.0
Nov					0		0.0
Dec					0		0.0
YTD	419,471	2,210,132	1,394,324	806,540	428,739	63.1%	
99 Average	208,465.17	144,875.42	61,998.00				
00 Average	212,409.58	151,979.25	62,324.00				
01 Average	268,423.58	168,145.98	95,583.64				
02 Average	293,211.60	190,499.94	103,537.15				
03 Average	315,606.48	197,041.87	116,546.74				
04 Average	315,733.14	199,189.14	115,220.00				

Dashboard Indicators

	YTD December 31		Year Ended September 30
	2004	2003	2002
Profitability Indicators (2):			
Operating Earnings	$1,693,800	$2,606,000	$1,146,600
% of Net Operating Revenue (Operating Margin)	2.3%	3.8%	1.9%
Nonoperating Gains	$324,000	$381,000	$230,000
Total Earnings	$2,017,800	$2,987,000	$1,376,600
% of Total Net Revenue (Excess Margin)	2.7%	4.3%	2.3%
EBITDA (1)	$5,811,800	$6,128,800	$4,013,200
% of Total Net Revenue	7.8%	8.9%	6.6%
Return on Assets	3.9%	6.1%	3.1%
Charity Care (% of Gross Charges)	1.3%	1.1%	1.1%
Volume Indicators (2):			
Unique Patients	36,020	36,100	36,430
WRVUs	313,520	297,420	274,920
Patient Encounters	178,570	175,900	173,760
Efficiency Indicators:			
WRVUs per Physician FTE	3.40%	3.50%	−1.8%
Revenue per WRVU Relative to Cost (2)	−1.97%	2.42%	−0.3%
Total Cost Per WRVU (3)	$215	$203	$197
% Change in Total Cost per WRVU from Prior Period	5.8%		
Salaries, Wages, and Benefits per WRVU (3)	$159	$156	$152
Liquidity Indicators:			
Days Cash on Hand (2)	74	65	59
Days in Receivables (3)(4)	48.6	46.6	47.0
Capital Structure Indicators:			
Debt to Capital (3)	46.3	49.1	52.9
Debt Service Coverage Indicators (2):			
Debt Service Coverage–Master Indenture	4.5	4.8	3.3
Debt Service Coverage–S&P*	3.5	3.8	2.5
Payer Mix (Based on Practice Charges):			
Fee for Service–Non-Medicare	35.6%	36.6%	38.2%
Health Plan	7.6%	7.8%	8.3%
Clinic Group	3.2%	3.1%	3.1%
Medicare	35.6%	34.8%	34.7%

Dashboard Indicators (continued)

	YTD December 31 2004	2003	Year Ended September 30 2002
Payer Mix (Based on Practice Charges):			
Medicaid	10.9%	10.2%	8.6%
PHP	1.3%	1.3%	1.1%
Other**	5.9%	6.1%	6.0%
Recovery by Payer			
Fee for Service–Non-Medicare	88.3%	88.1%	87.1%
Health Plan	80.1%	84.1%	77.9%
Clinic Group	56.5%	57.8%	59.0%
Medicare	35.3%	35.1%	38.3%
Medicaid	43.1%	43.9%	44.4%
PHP	39.5%	37.8%	44.1%
Other**	92.6%	92.5%	93.5%
Total All Payers	62.6%	63.7%	64.8%
Net Earnings from Operations	1,693,800	2,606,000	
Nonoperating Gains	324,000	381,000	
Net Earnings Before			
Extraordinary Items	2,017,800	2,987,000	
Depreciation and Amortization	2,816,200	2,376,600	
Interest	977,800	765,200	
Total Operating Revenue	74,823,800	69,089,000	
Total Assets	51,713,300	49,081,400	
Gross Charges	99,979,750	90,149,170	
Charity Care	1,288,330	987,960	
Total Assets	48,731,400	45,261,000	
Fiscal Period	1	1	

APPENDIX 5.3 INCOME DISTRIBUTION LEVELS

Compensation Formula with Allocation by 100% Productivity
January 1 Through December 31, 20XX

		Doctor A	Doctor B	Doctor C	Doctor D	Doctor E	Doctor F	Total
RVUs		8,318	6,727	4,889	4,197	8,325	6,634	39,090
Production %		21.28%	17.21%	12.51%	10.74%	21.30%	16.97%	100.00%
Receipts								
Based on Production	100%	574,563	464,613	337,698	289,881	575,035	458,209	2,700,000
Expenses								
Based on Production	40%	319,202	258,118	187,610	161,045	319,464	254,561	1,500,000
Net Income Distributable		255,362	206,495	150,088	128,836	255,571	203,649	1,200,000
Physician Compensation and Expenses								
Compensation		180,000	170,000	105,000	72,000	180,000	150,000	857,000
Profit Sharing		5,400	5,100	3,150	2,160	5,400	4,500	25,710
401(k) Match		5,400	5,100	3,150	2,160	5,400	4,500	25,710
Other Expenses		1,700	3,200	4,300	1,500	2,400	2,000	15,100
Payroll Taxes		8,190	8,045	7,103	5,508	8,190	7,755	44,791
Transcription Expense		12,000	5,000	400	4,600	9,000	8,000	39,000
Health Insurance		9,000	9,000	—	9,000	9,000	9,000	45,000
Disability		135	135	135	95	135	135	770
Continuing Education		10,100	3,300	1,100	800	4,000	3,500	22,800
Total Directly Identified Expenses		231,925	208,880	124,338	97,823	223,525	189,390	1,075,881
Distribution		23,437	(2,385)	25,750	31,013	32,046	14,259	124,119

Receipts and all overhead expenses are allocated based on the number of RVUs produced by the physician under the belief that those who produce more use more resources.

Compensation Formula with Allocation by Productivity and Equal Split
January 1 through December 31, 20XX

		Doctor A	Doctor B	Doctor C	Doctor D	Doctor E	Doctor F	Total
RVUs		8,318.42	6,726.57	4,889.12	4,196.85	8,325.25	6,633.86	39,090.06
Production		21.28%	17.21%	12.51%	10.74%	21.30%	16.97%	100.00%
Equal		16.67%	16.67%	16.67%	16.67%	16.67%	16.67%	100.00%
Receipts								
Split Equally	20%	90,000	90,000	90,000	90,000	90,000	90,000	540,000
Based on Production	80%	459,651	371,690	270,158	231,905	460,028	366,567	2,160,000
Total Allocable Receipts		549,651	461,690	360,158	321,905	550,028	456,567	2,700,000
Expenses								
Split Equally	60%	150,000	150,000	150,000	150,000	150,000	150,000	900,000
Based on Production	40%	127,681	103,247	75,044	64,418	127,786	101,824	600,000
Total Allocable Expenses		277,681	253,247	225,044	214,418	277,786	251,824	1,500,000
Net Income Distributable		271,970	208,443	135,114	107,487	272,243	204,743	1,200,000
Physician Compensation and Expenses								
Compensation		180,000	170,000	105,000	72,000	180,000	150,000	857,000
Profit Sharing		5,400	5,100	3,150	2,160	5,400	4,500	25,710
401(k) Match		5,400	5,100	3,150	2,160	5,400	4,500	25,710
Other Expenses Directly Identified		1,700	3,200	4,300	1,500	2,400	2,000	15,100
Payroll Taxes		8,190	8,045	7,103	5,508	8,190	7,755	44,791
Transcription Expense		12,000	5,000	400	4,600	9,000	8,000	39,000
Health Insurance		9,000	9,000	—	9,000	9,000	9,000	45,000
Disability		135	135	135	95	135	135	770
Continuing Education		10,100	3,300	1,100	800	4,000	3,500	22,800
Total Directly Identified Expenses		231,925	208,880	124,338	97,823	223,525	189,390	1,075,881
Distribution		40,045	(437)	10,777	9,664	48,718	15,353	124,119

This method is used to encourage some teamwork by sharing 20 percent of the revenue equally and to recognize that all physicians share on-call duties equally. Overhead expenses are allocated 40 percent production based RVUs and 60 percent equal based on the belief that 60 percent of the overhead is a fixed cost.

Compensation Formula with Net Income Allocation by Productivity and Equal Split
January 1 through December 31, 20XX

		Doctor A	Doctor B	Doctor C	Doctor D	Doctor E	Doctor F	Total
RVUs		8,318	6,727	4,889	4,197	8,325	6,634	39,090
Production %		21.28%	17.21%	12.51%	10.74%	21.30%	16.97%	100.00%
Equal %		16.67%	16.67%	16.67%	16.67%	16.67%	16.67%	100.00%
Split Equally	20%	40,000	40,000	40,000	40,000	40,000	40,000	240,000
Based on Production	80%	204,289	165,196	120,070	103,069	204,457	162,919	960,000
Total Allocable Net Income		244,289	205,196	160,070	143,069	244,457	202,919	1,200,000
Physician Compensation and Expenses								
Compensation		180,000	170,000	105,000	72,000	180,000	150,000	857,000
Profit Sharing		5,400	5,100	3,150	2,160	5,400	4,500	25,710
401(k) Match		5,400	5,100	3,150	2,160	5,400	4,500	25,710
Other Expenses Directly Identified		1,700	3,200	4,300	1,500	2,400	2,000	15,100
Payroll Taxes		8,190	8,045	7,103	5,508	8,190	7,755	44,791
Transcription Expense		12,000	5,000	400	4,600	9,000	8,000	39,000
Health Insurance		9,000	9,000	—	9,000	9,000	9,000	45,000
Disability		135	135	135	95	135	135	770
Continuing Education		10,100	3,300	1,100	800	4,000	3,500	22,800
Total Directly Identified Expenses		231,925	208,880	124,338	97,823	223,525	189,390	1,075,881
Distribution		12,364	(3,684)	35,733	45,246	20,932	13,529	124,119

Similar to the previous example; however, the pool (receipts less expenses) is split 20 percent equal and 80 percent based on RVUs. Note how the high producer (Dr. A) makes less in the scenario than in the previous example.

APPENDIX 5.4 GEOGRAPHIC PRACTICE COST INDICES (GCPIS)

Carrier Number	Loc. Number	Locality Name	Work GPCI	PE GPCI	MP GPCI
00510	00	Alabama	1.000	0.870	0.779
00831	01	Alaska	1.670	1.670	1.670
00832	00	Arizona	1.000	0.978	1.090
00520	13	Arkansas	1.000	0.847	0.389
31146	26	Anaheim/Santa Ana, CA	1.037	1.184	0.955
31146	18	Los Angeles, CA	1.056	1.139	0.955
31140	03	Marin/Napa/Solano, CA	1.015	1.248	0.669
31140	07	Oakland/Berkeley, CA	1.041	1.235	0.669
31140	05	San Francisco, CA	1.068	1.458	0.669
31140	06	San Mateo, CA	1.048	1.432	0.663
31140	09	Santa Clara, CA	1.063	1.380	0.622
31146	17	Ventura, CA	1.028	1.125	0.763
31146	99	Rest of California*	1.007	1.034	0.740
31140	99	Rest of California*	1.007	1.034	0.740
00824	01	Colorado	1.000	0.992	0.821
00591	00	Connecticut	1.050	1.156	0.933
00902	01	Delaware	1.019	1.035	0.802
00903	01	DC + MD/VA Suburbs	1.050	1.166	0.917
00590	03	Ft. Lauderdale, FL	1.000	1.018	1.790
00590	04	Miami, FL	1.015	1.052	2.399
00590	99	Rest of Florida	1.000	0.946	1.268
00511	01	Atlanta, GA	1.006	1.059	0.951
00511	99	Rest of Geordia	1.000	0.892	0.951
00833	01	Hawaii/Guam	1.000	1.124	0.817
05130	00	Idaho	1.000	0.881	0.478
00952	16	Chicago, IL	1.028	1.092	1.832
00952	12	East St. Louis, IL	1.000	0.924	1.720
00952	15	Suburban Chicago, IL	1.006	1.071	1.648
00952	99	Rest of Illinois	1.000	0.889	1.175
00630	00	Indiana	1.000	0.922	0.459
00826	00	Iowa	1.000	0.876	0.593
00650	00	Kansas*	1.000	0.895	0.738
00740	04	Kansas*	1.000	0.895	0.738
00660	00	Kentucky	1.000	0.866	0.875
00528	01	New Orleans, LA	1.000	0.945	1.240
00528	99	Rest of Louisiana	1.000	0.870	1.066
31142	03	Southern Maine	1.000	0.999	0.652
31142	99	Rest of Maine	1.000	0.910	0.652
00901	01	Baltimore/Surrounding Counties, MD	1.021	1.038	0.931
00901	99	Rest of Maryland	1.000	0.972	0.767
31143	01	Metropolitan Boston, MA	1.041	1.239	0.803
31143	99	Rest of Massachusetts	1.010	1.129	0.803

00953	01	Detroit, MI	1.043	1.038	2.741
00953	99	Rest of Michigan	1.000	0.938	1.545
00954	00	Minnesota	1.000	0.974	0.431
00512	00	Mississippi	1.000	0.837	0.750
00740	02	Metropolitan Kansas City, MO	1.000	0.967	0.896
00523	01	Metropolitan St. Louis, MO	1.000	0.938	0.893
00740	99	Rest of Missouri*	1.000	0.825	0.842
00523	99	Rest of Missouri*	1.000	0.825	0.842
00751	01	Montana	1.000	0.876	0.815
00655	00	Nebraska	1.000	0.877	0.442
00834	00	Nevada	1.005	1.039	1.138
31144	40	New Hampshire	1.000	1.030	0.883
00805	01	Northern NJ	1.058	1.193	0.916
00805	99	Rest of New Jersey	1.029	1.110	0.916
00521	05	New Mexico	1.000	0.900	0.898
00803	01	Manhattan, NY	1.094	1.351	1.586
00803	02	NYC Suburbs/Long Island, NY	1.068	1.251	1.869
00803	03	Poughkeepsie/N. NYC Suburbs, NY	1.011	1.075	1.221
14330	04	Queens, NY	1.058	1.228	1.791
00801	99	Rest of New York	1.000	0.944	0.720
05535	00	North Carolina	1.000	0.931	0.618
00820	01	North Dakota	1.000	0.880	0.630
00883	00	Ohio	1.000	0.944	0.967
00522	00	Oklahoma	1.000	0.876	0.413
00835	01	Portland, OR	1.000	1.049	0.438
00835	99	Rest of Oregon	1.000	0.933	0.438
00865	01	Metropolitan Philadelphia, PA	1.023	1.092	1.400
00865	99	Rest of Pennsylvania	1.000	0.929	0.790
00973	20	Puerto Rico	1.000	0.712	0.268
00870	01	Rhode Island	1.017	1.065	0.896
00880	01	South Carolina	1.000	0.904	0.336
00820	02	South Dakota	1.000	0.878	0.385
05440	35	Tennessee	1.000	0.900	0.612
00900	31	Austin, TX	1.000	0.996	0.922
00900	20	Beaumont, TX	1.000	0.890	1.318
00900	09	Brazoria, TX	1.000	0.978	1.318
00900	11	Dallas, TX	1.010	1.065	0.996
00900	28	Ft. Worth, TX	1.000	0.981	0.996
00900	15	Galveston, TX	1.000	0.969	1.318
00900	18	Houston, TX	1.020	1.007	1.316
00900	99	Rest of Texas	1.000	0.880	1.047
00910	09	Utah	1.000	0.941	0.653
31145	50	Vermont	1.000	0.986	0.527
00973	50	Virgin Islands	1.000	1.023	1.003
00904	00	Virginia	1.000	0.938	0.540
00836	02	Seattle (King County), WA	1.005	1.100	0.803
00836	99	Rest of Washington	1.000	0.972	0.803
00884	16	West Virginia	1.000	0.850	1.462
00951	00	Wisconsin	1.000	0.929	0.865
00825	21	Wyoming	1.000	0.895	0.970

STAFFING AND STAFF MANAGEMENT

Joseph W. Mitylng

Learning Objectives

This chapter will enable the reader to:

- identify the variables to be considered by hospitals, physician groups, and physician group leadership when deciding to add a physician to the group;
- learn an analytical technique for benchmarking the number and types of support staff in the group, and how to evaluate the implications of the benchmark data;
- gain an understanding of physician compensation systems, distinctions between quantifiable and nonquantifiable work, and techniques for valuing each;
- learn the core steps in developing or modifying a physician compensation system;
- identify useful sources of comparative staff compensation information;
- appreciate the difference between development and evaluation objectives in performance appraisal;
- learn the importance of including structure as well as process or outcome measures in a performance appraisal, particularly in relation to physicians; and
- learn both issue-oriented and proactive techniques for dealing with conflict and establishing strong relationships with physicians and staff, with the ultimate goal of a strong group culture.

Chapter Purpose

This chapter provides insights into decisions to recruit, evaluate staffing levels, develop compensation systems, appraise performance and provide feedback, provide continuing education, and establish strong relationships with physicians and staff, all with the aim of developing a strong culture. Human resource management is critical to all organizations. This is especially true in physician organizations because the primary assets of the organization are people and their relationships—with each other and with patients.

Case in Point

Mary Wilson had reached the end of her first month as executive director of The Medical Group, an independent, 40-physician multispecialty practice that admits to the 350-bed Midwest Hospital. Mary listed the issues she had identified in her first get-acquainted meetings with the physicians and staff at The Medical Group.

- Dr. James White, president of The Medical Group, had just been elected the previous month. He was highly regarded by the members of the group as a clinician and for his leadership in other areas, but he was new to the responsibilities of leading the whole group. He noted that he was looking forward to working with Mary and the skills she was bringing to the team.
- Dr. White had also noted that some in the group were interested in adding specialists and new offices, but other members of the group were strongly opposed. Frank Messer, president of Midwest Hospital, saw The Medical Group as a major strength in competing with other area hospitals, and Dr. White wondered what would be required to justify hospital support for the new physicians.
- The current compensation system was based on paying each physician a percentage of the revenue collected for their services, but it was known that some physicians received a higher percentage of their revenue than others. Members of the group felt the current physician compensation system was unfair and needed to be changed.
- The physicians felt the overhead in the practice, particularly staff cost, was high, but even with that cost they felt that current staff were not doing what was required of them.
- Support staff members felt disconnected from the physicians and the practice. Many saw their work as "just a job," and several were looking for other positions.

Mary had realized in taking her position that the job would have challenges, but each of these areas looked to be a major one. What should Mary's first step be?

Staff Planning

The following section addresses the challenges faced by both hospitals and group practices when planning for and recruiting physicians. Some of the same challenges are faced when planning for and recruiting nonphysician staff for group practices.

Physician Staff Planning

Hospitals and physician groups face different needs in justifying support to recruit a new physician. The following points summarize the approaches used to date and sources of needed information relevant to the decisions to be made by a hospital or medical group.

Hospitals may be recruiting to add staff in an existing employed physician group. In that context if the group has the kind of leadership accountable for the financial performance of the group, the recruiting decision will be made by much the same process as that outlined below for an independent physician group. The group's leadership has to decide if the added revenue from a new physician's practice is likely to be enough to justify adding that physician's services and costs to the group.

Hospital Recruiting

Hospitals also support recruiting physicians who are going to be in private practice and not employed by the hospital. The hospital's recruiting support decision in these cases faces several potential challenges:

- board presentation and approval;
- medical staff support sufficient to deal with concerns that the hospital may just be recruiting competition for the present staff; and
- regulatory requirements that any hospital support be justified by unmet community needs (see Chapters 3 and 10).

In these cases hospital leadership requires more objective analysis.

There are several sources of physician demand measures; Simmons and Harris (2004) summarize 12 of these sources published since 1980. Major recent sources cited include:

- Council on Graduate Medical Education (2000): "Update on the Physician Workforce"
- Cooper, Getzen, and Laud (2003): "Economic Expansion Is a Major Determinant of Physician Supply and Utilization"
- Solucient, LLC (2003): *Physician Community Requirements in the 21st Century: The 2003 Physicians to Population Ratios*
- Weiner (2004): "Prepaid Group Practice Staffing and U.S. Physician Supply: Lessons for Workforce Policy"

The above sources reflect a number of challenges in using objective data:

- **Identifying the qualifying factors that make the data in the sources appropriate for a given situation**: The data in each report represent an average set of assumptions for the population surveyed. Areas with a higher percentage of insured patients, patients with higher incomes, or

Medicare-age patients will have a higher demand for care than the average population reflected in the data. A prepaid group practice will care for the needs of a population with fewer physicians per 100,000 population as it manages the care provided by primary care physicians and referrals to specialists.

- **Accurately assessing the present effective number of full-time equivalent (FTE) physicians in the competitive area**: To what extent are the numbers of FTE physicians reflected in the phone book or medical society membership roster? These sources typically include physicians in full-time practice, physicians in part-time practice, and physicians who are listed but effectively no longer in practice; on the other hand new physicians who have been recently hired may not be listed.

- **The changing practice of medicine**: The use of hospitalists and intensivists has reduced the time primary care physicians and specialists have to spend in the hospital, increasing the numbers of patients for whom they are able to provide care. In addition increased use of nonsurgical approaches to providing care is increasing the demand for medical specialists and reducing the demand for surgeons.

Despite the challenges the objective data from these surveys and analyses—and the associated range of need estimates—provide a framework for addressing the concerns of the hospital board, members of the medical staff, and regulators.

Physician Group Recruiting

A physician group looks at recruiting a new physician from the standpoint of the costs and benefits to the practice of adding a new physician. When a new physician is first hired, the group has to pay the salary, benefits, and added support staff costs out of its revenue. If the practice needs to add another physician to care for the patients who come to the practice for care, the practice will grow and the new physician will be a net financial benefit to the practice as well as the incomes of the individual physicians. The physician group must answer three critical questions: Do we need to add another member to the group? Is it necessary that we add another physician at this time? Can this addition be justified by demand or the need for a new service?

Physician groups may find demographic patient demand analysis to be of value in deciding to recruit a new specialty. More often the group decides on the basis of the knowledge it has of the local medical community and the need for an added specialist in the community to meet the needs first of its existing patients and then of other patients seeking that specialty. For example, a primary care practice (family practice, internal medicine, and pediatrics) will have a good idea of the need for an added gastroenterologist in the community. Members of the group will know the ease or difficulty they have in referring patients to the existing gastroenterologists, the group will know who may be retiring and of planned additions to existing gastroenterology practices, and the group can estimate the volume of referrals the group itself generates that would support adding a gastroenterologist to it.

In recruiting members to physician specialties already in the group, the group looks at the burden on current members of the specialty in caring for the patients coming to the group for care. In private practice, in which the physician members are responsible for the added cost of the new physician, members of that specialty will often work harder than they would prefer to in order to expand the practice before adding a new physician. This will provide the new physician with a ready-made practice to step into and reduce the time it will take her to build a practice large enough to cover the added costs. The existing physicians will see a reduction in their salary to pay for the new physician while that physician builds her practice, but the new physician will also provide some immediate offsetting benefits, sharing the patient load, call, and eventually office overhead.

A physician group should consider several measures in deciding to recruit:

- **Time to next available appointment**: How long will people wait for this specialty? Patients may be willing to schedule an annual physical months in advance, but if they need to see an oncologist for the first time, they need to be seen immediately. Staff scheduling appointments—and physicians faced with the challenges of working patients in—will know if the group is turning away patients because physicians do not have enough time to provide timely appointments.

- **Perception of the present physicians looking to add a colleague**: If the current workload is more than the physicians want, and they are willing to see their incomes drop as the new colleague absorbs, at least initially, some of their patient volume (private practice reality), a physician group has the justification it needs to recruit.

- **Perception of the group's leadership**: If the group's leadership sees that the group has an opportunity to add a physician or new service that within a reasonable time will be financially self-supporting, better serve its patients, and build or strengthen the practice, leadership will develop that case for the group as a whole to support recruitment.

- **A physician group's first-hand knowledge of its market**: The opportunities and competition in a group's service area are the primary drivers in its decisions to recruit a new physician. Ratios of specialists per 100,000 people in the service area can provide guidance, but no arithmetic model can replace leadership judgment as to the number of patients who will choose this practice and number of referring physicians who will refer to this new specialist (see Box 6.1).

BOX 2.1

> The Marshfield Clinic in 1984 saw what it thought was an opportunity to re-cruit the first retinal surgeon at Marshfield Clinic. Marshfield is 15 miles from the geographic center of Wisconsin, and the only other retinal surgeons in Wisconsin at the time were in Madison and Milwaukee. The group's referrals alone were not enough to justify adding the specialty, but the clinic draws pa-tients from a wide area, and the decision was to recruit. In the first six months of practice the new retinal surgeon saw patients from Green Bay (east), Ash-land (north), Hudson (west), and just north of Madison (south). The retinal surgery practice proved to be successful.

Support Staff Planning

The cost survey published annually by the Medical Group Management As-sociation (MGMA 2004) provides a guide to appropriate staffing and staff compensation in medical groups. Deciding the best staffing for a specific group situation requires a review of current workflow to identify how to best use staff and make the decision to add or reduce staff or change present staff responsibilities. Determining appropriate staff compensation requires an analysis of the local market and compensation levels in that market, as will be discussed later in the chapter.

MGMA Cost Survey
Tables 6.1 and 6.2 show detailed staffing level information available in the MGMA cost survey (2004); the data are for single-specialty family practice groups, not hospital owned. Using the medians shown, practice management has a reference point to begin answering the questions of whether the group is staffing and paying appropriately.

Qualifiers
These data are provided on a voluntary basis by managers who are members of MGMA, and those responding to the survey do not always provide all of the detailed information shown. The median value for each line in Tables 6.1 and 6.2 is the midpoint of the responses for that line—half are above that value, and half are below. Any group is likely to be above the midpoint in one line and below the midpoint in another, so the detail is unlikely to add ex-actly to the totals. The differences between the median total reported does not equal the sum of the detail total, and the difference shown is typical. The data as shown do provide an indicator of the relative staffing of one position as compared to the others. This is the value of this survey report, a guide to trigger questioning of current staffing levels. The hard work of examining and evaluating present staff responsibilities, staffing levels, and practice cost to perform the various staff functions in a medical group will answer the question of what staffing should be.

Employee Category	% of Practice Revenue	
	Number Reporting	Median % Reported
Total Support Staff Cost	60	31.94
Total Employee Support Staff Salaries	54	26.00
General Administrative	55	2.91
Patient Accounting	55	3.49
General Accounting	31	.79
Managed Care, Administrative	16	.86
Information Technology	14	1.04
Housekeeping, Maintenance, Security	10	.69
Medical Receptionists	53	4.59
Medical Secretaries, Transcriptionists	32	1.31
Medical Records	47	1.63
Other Administrative Support	22	.47
Registered Nurses	40	2.67
Licensed Practical Nurses	42	2.38
Medical Assistants, Nurses Aides	53	4.02
Clinical Laboratory	34	2.10
Radiology and Imaging	30	1.21
Other Medical Support Services	16	.87
Total Employee Staff Benefits	58	5.71
Total Contracted Support Staff	19	.38
Total of Detail Subtotals*		32.09

TABLE 6.1
Staff Cost as Percentage of Practice Revenue

* Sum of total employee support staff salaries, total employee staff benefits, and total contracted support staff.

SOURCE: MGMA 2004.

The total reported is typically the most reliable median value because it is based on the largest number of responses. Some managers reporting their data only provide the information at the total level and do not bother with the detail. In other cases groups may not have a specific cost such as housekeeping as part of their practice costs, as it may be included in the rent.

Those who wish to can normalize the detailed data so the sum of the median data detail equals the total reported median. It is important to remember that the purpose of these data is to obtain and present useful insights into how other groups spend their staffing dollars. Ordinarily it would be expected that the sum of the detail percentages would equal the total reported percentage of revenue cost for staff. Recognizing that the median values shown for each detail item in Tables 6.1 and 6.2 collectively do not represent any one practice, the median values shown for each detail item can be proportionately

Normalizing the data

TABLE 6.2
Staff FTEs per
FTE Provider

Employee Category	FTEs per Physician	
	Number Reporting	Median Reported
Total Support Staff Cost	60	31.94
Total Employee Support Staff per FTE Provider	43	3.50
General Administrative	37	.19
Patient Accounting	37	.52
General Accounting	21	.09
Managed Care, Administrative	10	.11
Information Technology	11	.13
Housekeeping, Maintenance, Security	5	*
Medical Receptionists	36	.80
Medical Secretaries, Transcriptionists	24	.20
Medical Records	32	.31
Other Administrative Support	15	.07
Registered Nurses	26	.34
Licensed Practical Nurses	31	.38
Medical Assistants, Nurses Aides	36	.68
Clinical Laboratory	21	.27
Radiology and Imaging	21	.13
Other Medical Support Services	11	.14
Total Contracted Support Staff	4	*
Detail Total		4.36

*Number of responses is too low.

SOURCE: MGMA 2004.

adjusted if that is helpful in using the data. The sum of the detail will equal the total reported, as shown in Table 6.3.

Median values should not be the goal

The MGMA Survey of Better Performing Practices showed that better-performing practices have more staff than the median, not less. It is also true that some poorer-performing practices have more staff. The better-performing practices make better use of their staff to support income-producing ancillary services (e.g., lab, x-ray, and EKG testing) or to make the physicians and other income-producing staff more productive. The poorer-performing practices just have more staff; the potential benefits of having more staff are not being realized.

Mastering Patient Flow

Survey data can be a guide to questioning the group's current staffing level, as noted above: If the median is X, why are we so different from X? Answering the question of what the group's staffing should be, however, requires understanding how staff are presently being used and identifying any changes

TABLE 6.3
Normalized Staff Cost as Percentage of Practice Revenue

Employee Category	% of Practice Revenue		Normalized Subtotal	Normalized Detail %
	Number Reporting	Median % Reported	Adjusted Subtotal Median % to Total	Adjusted Detail Median % to Adjusted Subtotals
Total Support Staff Cost	60	31.94	31.94	31.94
Total Employee Support Staff Salaries	54	26.00	25.88	25.88
General Administrative	55	2.91		2.43
Patient Accounting	55	3.49		2.91
General Accounting	31	.79		.66
Managed Care, Administrative	16	.86		.72
Information Technology	14	1.04		.87
Housekeeping, Maintenance, Security	10	.69		.58
Medical Receptionists	53	4.59		3.83
Medical Secretaries, Transcriptionists	32	1.31		1.09
Medical Records	47	1.63		1.36
Other Administrative Support	22	.47		.39
Registered Nurses	40	2.67		2.23
Licensed Practical Nurses	42	2.38		1.98
Medical Assistants, Nurses Aides	53	4.02		3.35
Clinical Laboratory	34	2.10		1.75
Radiology and Imaging	30	1.21		1.01
Other Medical Support Services	16	.87		.73
Total Employee Staff Benefits	58	5.71	5.68	5.68
Total Contracted Support Staff	19	.38	.38	.38
Subtotal Detail Total		32.09	31.94	31.94

SOURCE: MGMA 2004.

that will make better use of staff, improve practice performance and profitability, or reduce the practice's staff cost.

In every practice staff have been added over time as seemed to be required by the specific practice. With passing time the staffing and duties of each position come to be seen as the givens in a practice. The interpersonal relationships that develop tend to cement those positions in place. But is the current staffing what it should be?

Triage nurses were added to meet the needs for less-costly care under capitation, a fixed amount of reimbursement per patient per month. Triage nurses answer patients' questions over the phone, when they can, and avoid the need for an office visit. Triage nurses are highly skilled and, although paid less than physicians, are well paid. Although payer reimbursement has shifted away from capitation and back to fee-for-service reimbursement, many practices still employ triage nurses. The practice is no longer paid by capitation for most of its patients, and there is no revenue to pay for the triage nurse's care for fee-for-service patients. The work of the nurse negates the need for the patient to come in for an appointment, and the physician cannot bill for that care. The question is what the physician group's staffing should be today.

Woodcock (2003) outlines an approach to identifying ways to better organize workflow and in so doing make better use of staff. The key concept is that physician time and the time of nurse practitioners, physician assistants, and others who can bill for their services is the most valuable resource in the practice. The key to success is in maximizing the productive (billable) use of physician time. Woodcock (referring to physician time as the time of all billable providers) notes: "Physicians' time can be divided into three categories: productive, wasted and delegated. The key to success is to maximize the productive time, eliminate the wasted time and hire support staff to handle what can be delegated" (Woodcock 2003, p. 11).

Compensation and Benefit Programs

The following sections describe approaches to developing, reviewing, and managing compensation and benefit programs for physicians and support staff.

Physician Compensation and Benefits

The goal of a physician compensation system is to reward the physician members of the group in such a way that each member of the group feels reasonably rewarded for the work he does.

An Equitable System?   A senior physician at Virginia Mason Clinic in Seattle observed several years ago: "There is no such thing as an 'equitable' physician compensation system; the best you can hope to do is an 'acceptable' compensation system."

The wisdom in this observation is the recognition that the work physicians do is varied and cannot be measured on a single scale. Caring for patients is a core work requirement in most groups, and it can be readily valued by the cash collected for that work, or by the relative value units (RVUs) of work done. But other valuable work is not so easily measured. How do you recognize the value of the senior physician who is widely known in the community and is a major reason new patients come to the group for care? How do you value the physician who is the "doctor's doctor" in the group, the one other physicians seek out for advice in caring for particularly difficult cases?

The challenge in developing a compensation system is to find ways to appropriately reward individuals for the varied work they do. The most that can be accomplished is to develop an acceptable system, a system in which individual physicians feel they are being paid fairly for what they do.

Part of the fairness assessment is external. The following surveys, published annually, show the relationship between compensation and production for many specialists who practice in single- and multispecialty groups, by region and nationally:

- Physician Compensation and Production Survey (MGMA 2004)
- Medical Group Compensation & Financial Survey (American Medical Group Association and RSM McGladrey 2004)

A significant part of the perceived fairness in a group, though, is the perception of internal fairness. The rest of this section describes a process to develop individual compensation that is seen to be fair internally.

Some groups have compensation systems that are stable for periods of several years. This is particularly true in groups with a strong culture in which individual physicians find value in being part of the group. These physicians know they are not interested in leaving the group, they are less likely to pay attention to what compensation might be in a different group, and the physicians as a group are not interested in changing the system until a majority of the group sees a significant problem with it. The disruption in the group caused by a system change is not worth the effort otherwise.

In contrast many groups are said to have three systems: the system they had last year, the system they have this year, and the system they will have next year. When individual compensation is seen as the primary value of being a member of the group, individuals may choose to seek to change the compensation system or leave the group.

Much effort has gone into measuring the value of the work performed by each member of the group, both quantifiable and nonquantifiable. Some work can be measured by objective measures such as dollars collected or RVUs; other work requires subjective measures such as the assessment of the group's leadership and the degree to which an individual serves the group through committee work, research, or education.

Measures of Quantifiable and Nonquantifiable Work

Table 6.4 shows common measures of quantifiable work and the strengths and weaknesses of each.

Physician groups deal with nonquantifiable work in two ways: summary decisions that are applied to individuals, and measurements that attempt to quantify the judgments of colleagues and patients as a way of measuring performance in these inherently nonquantifiable areas.

Examples of summary decisions include:

- "Everyone does their share": Taking call is an example. There is no special compensation because everyone does their share. An often-seen corollary, though, is a reduction in compensation if someone chooses to opt out of call.
- "Someone does more": Taking the responsibility of being president of the group is an example. A value is placed on the individual's time devoted to the activity. In some cases the value is the calculated as value of the time taken from clinical work; in other cases it is a fixed amount for the position regardless of who fills it.

Examples of measures to quantify the judgments of patients, colleagues, and staff include:

- Colleague and staff surveys: Colleagues and staff can be surveyed in relatively simple ways such as a five-question survey that asks for feedback on a scale of one to five about questions such as an individual's collegiality (handling their own responsibilities and being responsive to requests for help by others). The leader who meets with physicians to review each individual's performance will have the responses summarized and review the summary with each individual.
- Patient satisfaction surveys: Many hospitals and integrated delivery systems use Press-Ganey for patient satisfaction measures (Press-Ganey and Associates 2005).

On the clinical side quality-of-life instruments have been developed to measure patients' activities related to living with chronic disease as well as patients' pre- and postsurgery activities.

Developing or Modifying a Compensation System

It is important to involve a broad, representative base of physicians. The process may include all physicians in smaller groups and a broad base of formal and informal leaders in larger groups. In determining the size of the group the objective is to make it large enough to be seen by the group as reasonably inclusive but not so large as to be unable to discuss the issues. In all groups the active involvement of leadership is critical to working through the trade-offs to deal simultaneously with the interests of individuals and the group.

Compensation plan objectives

The first task is to discuss how the individuals see the group and agree on the objectives for the compensation plan. At one extreme the group sees itself as

Measure	Strengths	Weaknesses
Gross Charges	A measure of work volume	Depends on charge level, which may be heavily discounted by payers; not cash collected
Collected Revenue	A measure of work volume and cash collected—direct value to the group	Focuses on revenue only and affected by the variation in payment levels between well-insured care and indigent care; also, the net value to group may be largely offset by costs in generating the revenue (e.g., collections and costs for oncology drugs and immunizations)
Work Relative Value Units (wRVUs)	A measure of work volume that is independent of the variation in payer reimbursement levels; the purest measure of individual work; converted to collections credit by an average conversion factor across all payers; a good way of measuring work in a compensation system	RVUs are not cash; rewarding on the basis of wRVUs will reward the development of a low- or nonpaying practice, which can be a reasonable objective for a practice with a mission to care for indigent patients; does not measure the revenues or costs involved in providing the care
Revenue Minus Expenses	A measure of net cash value of the work to the group; provides incentive for physicians paid on this net cash value to identify ways to both increase practice revenue and decrease costs	Tends to focus individual physicians on their individual financial performance and use of practice expenses; group leadership must find ways to value low- or nonpaying work outside of revenue collected to provide an incentive to do this work

TABLE 6.4
Strengths and Weaknesses of Various Measures of Production

a collection of individual practices that only practice together for their individual convenience. Such a group is often described as a group in name only, and maximizing individual compensation for the work done is the objective. At the other extreme individuals want to be paid at reasonably competitive levels, but investing in the group and ensuring its long-term growth and development are important objectives also. In all groups the objectives of individuals fall along this spectrum, but the core of a stable group will have similar objectives. An individual whose personal objectives differ significantly from the rest of the group will—and should—eventually choose to leave the group.

Decide what to value

It is in the process of deciding what to value that the objectives of individuals are evident. The compensation plan can reward people for any or all of the following:

- Production
- Production adjusted for practice expenses
- Quality
- Collegiality
- Seniority
- Practice development ("rainmaker")
- Leadership
- Administrative time
- Teaching time
- Research

After a discussion of what is included in each item and how each item would be measured, the items can be listed and the group votes first on the items to be included in the plan.

Assign relative weights that total to 100 percent of calculated compensation

When the items to be rewarded have been identified, the second step is to vote on the percentage weight to be applied to each item. The percentage weight is the percentage of the total amount available for physician compensation that goes into a compensation pool for a given item for the group. For example, if the compensation pool were $500,000 and the group decided that 80 percent of the compensation pool should be distributed on the basis of production, $400,000 would be distributed among the physicians in the group proportional to their individual production as shown in Table 6.5.

Show individuals what the new compensation system will mean for their compensation based on their present level of work

In addition to the production-based compensation, the group may have decided to pay Dr. Smith a stipend of $10,000 for his work as the leader of the group and to divide the rest of the compensation pool equally. That produces total compensation for each individual as shown in Table 6.6.

Individuals need to know how their compensation will be affected by a new system. Producing tables such as the above based on each individual's actual production and the actual compensation pool for the group will show each individual what her compensation would be under the proposed new system.

TABLE 6.5
Production-based Compensation

Physician	Individual Production	Production-based Compensation
Dr. Smith	$ 250,000	$ 100,000
Dr. Jones	$ 250,000	$ 100,000
Dr. Wilson	$ 500,000	$ 200,000
Total	$ 1,000,000	$ 400,000

Physician	Production Compensation	Leadership Compensation	Equal Share Compensation	Total Compensation
Dr. Smith	$100,000	$10,000	$30,000	$140,000
Dr. Jones	$100,000		$30,000	$130,000
Dr. Wilson	$200,000		$30,000	$230,000
Total	$400,000	$10,000	$90,000	$500,000

TABLE 6.6

Production and Other Factors Leading to Total Compensation

In the example in Table 6.6 the current system (the one the group is operating under before the change to pay an amount to the leader and some equal share) may be one of 100 percent productivity. Dr. Wilson may have realized that some of his production is due to the leadership of Dr. Smith and the patients that Drs. Smith and Jones attract to the practice. Dr. Wilson may have suggested the group look at a change in the compensation system to more fairly reward Drs. Smith and Jones for their contributions to the practice (and keep the group and his referrals together). Table 6.7 shows each individual what he would receive under the new compensation system compared to the present system.

Table 6.7 illustrates the point made earlier: "There is no such thing as an 'equitable' compensation system; the best you can hope to achieve is an 'acceptable' compensation system." Depending on the relationship between the three physicians as well as the practice situation, Dr. Wilson may decide the new compensation system is totally unacceptable or reasonable and acceptable.

If the size of the change for individuals is potentially large, one step to achieving an acceptable system change is to phase in the change over six to 18 months (see Table 6.8).

The phase-in time will give individuals whose compensation is likely to drop time to change their performance and potentially maintain or increase their salaries under the new system.

Under the draw system, compensation is paid as a guaranteed monthly salary, or draw, for the year; payments are made at a level the group can expect to support for the year. To continue with the example in Table 6.8 the group

Reach agreement on a compensation system that will meet the needs of the organization and be reasonably acceptable to most physicians

Bonuses

Physician	Current 100% Production System	Proposed New System	Difference
Dr. Smith	$ 125,000	$ 140,000	+$ 15,000
Dr. Jones	$ 125,000	$ 130,000	+$ 5,000
Dr. Wilson	$ 250,000	$ 230,000	–$ 20,000
Total	$ 500,000	$ 500,000	0

TABLE 6.7

Comparison of 100 Percent Production Versus a New System Based on Priorities

Period of Phase-in	Old System Weight	New System Weight
First six months	2/3	1/3
Second six months	1/2	1/2
Third six months	1/3	2/3
After 18 months	0	100%

may decide that the practice volume varies little from month to month, but the group wants to have an amount in reserve to be sure they have enough to pay expenses from month to month. The payers may decide to delay payments for a month, but the monthly expenses still have to be paid.

The above salaries under the new system would be reduced to 80 percent of the projected salaries for each individual, as shown in Table 6.9, and paid monthly based on that level.

At the end of the year the production of each individual may have been exactly the same as projected, but due to a reduction in practice costs during the year there is $10,000 more in the pool than anticipated. After paying 100 percent of the projected compensation, the physician compensation pool has $10,000 remaining to be distributed to the members of the group.

Bonuses are paid to individuals from the dollars left at year end. The questions of who decides on the individual bonus amounts and the criteria for deciding the amounts by individual are the final points to be decided.

Physician benefits

The compensation referenced above is salary and bonus compensation and gets most of the attention. For relatively high-income individuals, however, added benefits that are seen as valuable and paid for with pretax dollars are worth more than the same dollars paid as taxable income.

Benefits provided and the cost of the benefits are paid before the calculation of the dollars available for the compensation pool. The cost of the benefits is a direct trade-off with the dollars available for compensation. In a smaller group, the group as a whole will decide the benefits to be paid by the group. Larger groups find it useful to establish a compensation and benefits committee to do the work of exploring possible new benefits and recommending changes for the group to consider.

Physician	Projected Compensation	80% Draw
Dr. Smith	$140,000	$112,000
Dr. Jones	$130,000	$104,000
Dr. Wilson	$230,000	$184,000
Total	$500,000	$400,000

Support Staff Compensation and Benefits

It is important to perform surveys of salaries and benefits for similar positions in the local area. Turnover is expensive, and hearing about significant salary differences for staff as someone gives notice that they are leaving is an expensive way to learn about competitive salaries in the community.

Compensation

In place of regular surveys smaller physician groups learn about competitive salaries from the information gathered in the process of replacing individuals who leave. Some turnover typically occurs in a medical group as a result of people moving from the area, going back to school, and other unavoidable reasons for staff to leave the practice. The process of recruiting replacements to fill open positions provides a first-hand opportunity to learn what candidates are looking at as competitive positions and compensation in the community. Persuading good candidates to consider a position requires a reasonably competitive compensation structure. Candidates who are seriously looking at a position will often say they are looking at another position and mention the salary offered. If the salary quoted appears unrealistic, that is a signal to survey competitive positions and the salaries offered for those positions. When receptionist candidates are turning down positions to take check-out positions in the local supermarket, there is a strong indication that the group's current salary level for receptionists is too low. The employers who make the competitive offers that good candidates accept and good employees leave for are the ones to survey.

Local hospital pay scales are a reference point, but it is important to consider differing job requirements. The hospital positions are still in health-care, but for the right candidates the opportunity to work with a physician in a smaller office setting is more desirable than a position with similar responsibilities in a large hospital. Physician groups cannot afford to match the salaries and benefits available to hospital staff; physician groups need to build on their other strengths to attract the best staff.

Benefits for staff are determined by what the physicians want to support and by what is required to attract and retain competent staff. In general staff benefits in a physician's office are much lower than the benefits for positions with comparable responsibilities in a hospital.

Benefits

One benefit area may be higher in a medical group: the contribution to a retirement plan. The Employee Retirement Income Security Act requires that the retirement benefits for lower-paid employees be reasonably consistent with the retirement benefits paid to higher-income employees. That requirement has led some physician groups to provide good retirement plans for their employees. Other physician groups have gone to the other extreme of providing no retirement plan within the group beyond a noncontributory 401(k), which is funded only by contributions by the employees. Higher-income employees, including the physicians, develop and fund their own retirement programs.

Performance Appraisal and Evaluation Systems

Performance appraisal and evaluation is too often seen as a burden—just paperwork that takes time and gets in the way of the real work of dealing with the issues that arise each day. An effective performance appraisal and evaluation system is integral to the effective management and leadership of a group. An effective process provides feedback to individuals on what they are doing well and what they could do better. An effective process also generates a dialogue with individuals on the barriers in the workplace that prevent them from doing their best work. Addressing those barriers provides the opportunity to eliminate them and often address at the same time the root causes of those issues that arise each day.

Objectives of Performance and Evaluation Systems

The objectives of performance and evaluation systems fall into two categories: the development of the individual and evaluation of the individual's performance against goals or the performance of others (Lyons and Callahan 1996). Development objectives include added training, education and work experiences, and goal setting that the individual and manager both see as worthy aspirations for personal improvement.

Evaluation reviews may be based on goals as well as the performance of others. For purposes of evaluation the goals are seen more in the light of expected performance by both the individual and the manager. They may be referred to as stretch goals, but both the individual and the manager see the goals as realistically being accomplished with a reasonable stretch.

Both sets of objectives are important. To keep a focus on the importance of each set, researchers have recommended that evaluation reviews be done when salary changes for the following year are discussed and that development reviews occur at a different time (Lyons and Callahan 1996).

Performance Appraisal Content

Avedis Donabedian, MD, MPH (1966), developed the concepts of structure, process, and outcome for evaluating the quality of healthcare:

- **Outcomes**: Results of the individual's work (e.g., number of patients seen, charges generated, and patient satisfaction for physicians; number of patients appointed, patient satisfaction with appointment time, and accuracy of medical record filing for staff).
- **Process**: How the individual does her work (e.g., timeliness of completing medical record notes and charge sheets and practicing evidence-based medicine for physicians; making appointments according to physician guidelines and timely filing of medical record information for staff).

- **Structure**: What are the barriers that limit individual performance? Examples of barriers include facilities, equipment, staffing, supplies, and operating procedures (workflow, how the work is done).

  Outcomes and process measures are the basis of evaluation reviews, and process measures are also the basis for development reviews. The following sections describe the importance of the explicit inclusion of structure in achieving performance improvement in medical groups.

Structure in Performance Improvement

Structural barriers are often brought up in discussing individual performance, particularly as a way to explain lower-than-expected performance, in both evaluation and development reviews. Including structure as an explicit consideration in a performance appraisal shifts the discussion from explaining and complaining to joint problem solving. The explicit consideration of structure has been found to be the key to real and sustainable improvement in performance.

In a four-year research project Lyons and Callahan (1996) worked with physicians in group practice and solo settings to use appraisals to improve medical care behaviors and outcomes. Their research produced some important findings:

1. The research "found consistent and pervasive improvement in care behaviors only when feedback on processes and outcomes was combined with intensive diagnostic and problem-solving activities regarding their organizational structures and situations. Feedback of traditional process and outcome data, without situational diagnoses and problem solving, was followed by **no** improvement in performance" (Lyons and Callahan 1996, p. 138).
2. The structural changes that came out of the situational diagnoses and action plans in many cases did not require additional budget or other resources. Some examples of these changes were: "creative and new reporting or recording procedures, correcting communication and coordination glitches between and within departments, reassignment of responsibilities, and improved use of existing education programs" (Lyons and Callahan 1996, p. 139).

Lyons and Callahan further found that the greatest improvements occurred when added time was devoted to following up on action plans to remove the barriers.

Physician Performance Appraisal

Physician performance appraisal is a weak area in most groups, and that weakness is understandable in a physician practice environment:

- Individual physicians see themselves as providing good medical care.
- Performance data are always seen as a report card evaluation.
- Data that show less-than-perfect performance are "bad data" until proven otherwise.

However developmentally a performance appraisal has been presented, physicians see performance appraisal as an evaluation. Physician performance appraisal has been a painful process for all involved and has become something to avoid.

Value of Structure Review

The approach of tying a review of structure into a process or outcome data review, as reported by Lyons and Callahan (1996), has significant advantages:

- It addresses first the real possibility of performance factors outside the physician's control.
- Identifying and addressing those factors builds physician buy-in for the process.
- The process is seen by physicians as providing value to them by helping them provide better care for their patients.

Value of Colleague Review

In preparation for a performance review the medical director may choose to develop a set of questions with the physicians to highlight any issues in the functioning of the group. This is a useful way of providing peer-group feedback on the performance of members in the group. Some examples of possible questions include whether an individual:

- helps finish the work at the end of the day;
- carries her share of the workload;
- works well with other physicians; and
- works well with staff.

The key is to engage the physicians in the group in developing the questions so they are seen as relevant to the performance of the group. Individual responses to the survey are tabulated outside the group, in the medical director's office, so the responses of individuals are not known by anyone in the group. Only the composite responses are presented back to the group, and any information that would tie a specific response back to an individual member of the group is deleted.

Value of 360-degree Review

A 360-degree review expands the review group to include physicians who may be customers of the group, leadership of the larger organization, and staff who work directly with the group of physicians. Expanding to include support staff as well as colleagues is a final stage in developing a strong practice group culture. In every group one or more physicians are in tune with the feelings of the staff. Those physicians will bring their concerns into the colleague review noted above. The inclusion of staff can evolve as an idea from the comments of colleagues, and the medical director can encourage that step when he judges the time is right.

The medical director initiates and leads the physician review process. In that process the medical director:

Responsibility of Medical Director

- provides feedback to individual physicians;
- arranges development opportunities for individual physicians; and
- engages administrative leadership to work with physicians in addressing the structural issues.

An effective medical director works closely with each physician, standing firm on reasonable performance expectations but being ready to understand and work with each physician to address structural issues limiting their performance. That stance is the essence of a medical director's firm but fair relationship with physicians.

Support Staff Performance Appraisal

Individual staff members, like physicians, can see the structural issues in their work. Consciously including a review of structural as well as process or outcome criteria in staff reviews will also pay dividends.

Staff performance reviews are typically undertaken by the staff supervisor. The supervisor talks with other staff and physicians who work with the individual to obtain their feedback. The supervisor completes the review forms, schedules a time to meet, and presents the review to the staff member.

It helps to give the employee a copy of the most recent prior review to have him consider the earlier performance goals that were agreed on and to develop the employee's assessment of what he has accomplished. Have supervisory and management staff prepare their own assessment of the prior year's performance and provide that self-assessment to their manager before the performance appraisal meeting. Even with the best intentions managers find themselves with a scheduled performance review and less time than they would like to prepare. In that situation a manager may overlook some good performance of the individual in the past year. That oversight will be avoided by giving the individual a chance to summarize what she has accomplished before the review.

New managers need to learn that the primary objective of the performance appraisal is not to list all the ways the individual might have performed better in the past year. If serious performance issues exist, those issues should be addressed as they arise with warnings and agreed-on action plans to improve performance.

The primary objective of the performance appraisal process is to review first what has been working well and celebrate those successes. The second objective is to talk about areas where the individual could do better in the future. An explicit discussion of any structural issues and what can be done to address them as part of improving future performance should be part of this second objective.

Employee Education Programs

Employee education can be done by paying for participation in external training programs sponsored by associations such as MGMA, by the local hospital or medical society, and by colleges. If the group is large enough, the program can be done in-house by the experts in the organization or by experts drawn from area academic programs.

Inhouse Programs Led by the Organization's Experts

Examples of common in-house programs include budgeting, reading revenue and expense reports, billing and collections, coding and compliance, and performance appraisal. Conducting in-house programs on these topics for people drawn from cross-functional areas builds awareness of the shared performance required by individuals in different work areas to achieve effective performance as an organization. In the billing and collections area, for example, what the front desk does in verifying insurance as patients come in for services does directly affect the billing office's ability to collect.

There is a significant advantage to using the organization's experts where the experts are reasonably comfortable in this role: It builds respect in the organization for its capabilities. The disadvantage to this approach is that it requires leadership to take the time to prepare, but the benefits typically outweigh this disadvantage for effective leaders.

Inhouse Programs Led by Outside Experts

Area academic programs and independent consultants are resources that can be drawn on to lead in-house programs on the topics noted above. Outside experts are particularly good for providing programs on topics related to building a stronger organization, such as a program on insights to be drawn from Jim Collin's (2001) book *Good to Great*. The use of outside presenters in this context also enables leadership to be part of the learning group.

Employee Relations and Conflict Resolution

It has been said that the resources of a medical group walk in during the morning and walk out at night. Those resources are bright, capable, responsible individuals with a spirit of independence and self-reliance. They expect to be able to state their ideas and have them heard and considered. In that context leading and managing the relationships between people, and resolving the inevitable conflicts that arise, is a continuing challenge. This section presents some ideas that leaders and managers can use to deal with that challenge.

Leadership Sets the Tone

Individuals in leadership roles set the tone for how people are expected to deal with one another. Conflicts arise in several sets of relationships:

- physicians dealing with physicians;
- physicians dealing with staff; and
- staff and physicians dealing with patients.

The movie *The Godfather* contains a line that many people remember: "Give 'em a deal they can't refuse." In the context of dealing with relationships in a medical group another line is the one to live by: "You gotta show respect!" In every context, showing respect for the individual and her views is the first requirement. Agreement cannot occur in every case, but leaders and managers need to show respect. Expecting respect in return is another key requirement.

Conflict Situations Provide Teachable Moments

Dealing with conflict in relationships is an inherent part of leading and managing a medical group, as noted. It is important to remember in that process that most people view dealing with conflict to be difficult. Conflict draws attention, and how a conflict is handled provides a teachable moment for the individuals involved and for the organization.

Conflicts challenge relationships, and the strength of a leadership team is in its ability to decide which member of the team has the best relationship and should address a particular issue. Regardless of the relationship the conflict must be addressed. Respect must be shown each individual in seeking to understand the views of all involved. There may be no good solution that meets the interests of each individual, but if each individual's views—including those in leadership—have been heard and respected in trying to find a solution, the individuals and the organization will see that the basic principle of showing respect for the individual has been honored.

Often there are ways to resolve conflicts that work reasonably well for all involved. Resolving conflicts successfully builds and strengthens relationships.

Proactive Meetings with Employees

A regular meeting of the administrator with groups of employees is a good way to minimize conflicts. The administrator meets with employees in groups of 25 to 50 people and provides an opportunity for individuals to be heard.

The meetings create a culture in which employees know that they and their views are respected.

There are three parts to these meetings:

1. **Informal presentation**: The meeting begins with a brief, informal presentation by the administrator that provides updates on major organizational activities (e.g., building program, adding new equipment, new initiatives with the hospital).

2. **Open forum**: Employees are able to ask the executive director or administrator whatever is of interest to them. Answering those questions as they come provides value in many ways. The value for individuals is that they feel "in the know" and respected. The value for the administrator is to learn of any issues that are brewing and correct any misunderstandings in an easy, informal way; the process builds tremendous credibility for the administrator with the employees. The value of the open forum for the organization is that it builds a culture in which individuals see the organization as open and respecting all individuals and their views. The process builds loyalty to the leadership and the organization.

3. **Follow-up**: A few questions may require some research to answer. The commitment is to get back to the group with an answer in a communication to all employees, and to send that communication as soon as the answer is known.

These meeting are held at least annually (every six months is better) and more often if major topics, like changes in health plan benefits, arise. The pattern of these meetings provides a powerful vehicle for talking directly with employees on all issues that affect them.

Proactive Meetings with Physicians and Other Clinical Providers

Regular meetings by the president and administrator with all physicians and other clinical providers have similar benefits in developing a culture of open communication. They may include all clinical providers in meetings with physicians, or the meetings with other clinical providers may need to be handled separately, but the basic meeting process of update, question and answer, and feedback is the same as outlined above.

These meetings occur in addition to the regular governance meetings with the group's board or executive committee. Depending on the physician group's comfort with the leadership and financial performance of the group, an executive summary of the board minutes may be sufficient. Individuals can contact the president or administrator if there are points on which they want additional information.

If the group is undergoing major change or its financial performance is in question, monthly meetings to which all physicians are invited will be well-attended. The basic format of update, question and answer, and feedback works well in this setting also. The willingness to take all questions and answer them candidly builds credibility in these meetings.

An annual meeting with all physicians and spouses is valuable and expected in medical groups. This provides a chance to review the performance of the previous year and celebrate the successes, new staff, and retiring staff.

The Result: A Strong Group Culture

The net effect of these meetings is a culture in which the belief held by the members of the group and staff is that: "We can talk about and resolve any issue." The human relations staff, in its dealing with employees and physicians, reinforces the group culture of a team that respects and values one another.

Individuals who are treated in this way know the organization's leadership respects and values them; they respond by respecting and valuing the leaders. Individuals who are treated in this way see the organization as a good place to work and a good place for care; they tell people they know, and they recruit new employees and patients.

Summary

The decisions to recruit physicians and staff are the most expensive decisions in a physician group. Staffing and paying appropriately are critical to the financial success and stability of the group, but so is the ability to perform effective performance appraisals and provide appropriate feedback. This chapter provides insights into what is required in each of these areas. The final section outlines some steps for dealing with issue-oriented conflict and steps that leaders and managers can take to develop strong relationships with physicians and staff, with the ultimate goal of developing a strong group culture.

Discussion Questions

1. Why is it important for a group's physicians to be involved in deciding whether to add another physician in their specialty?
2. Why might a leadership group decide to add a physician in a specialty even though the physicians in that specialty do not see the need? What steps might leadership take to make the physicians in the specialty at least neutral regarding adding a colleague?
3. Why is it important to value both quantifiable and nonquantifiable work in the compensation plan? What will make it necessary to value both?
4. Why is it particularly important to include structure as well as process and outcomes in the performance appraisal process for physicians?

5. Describe two keys to success in dealing with conflicts.
6. Describe some proactive approaches that leadership can take to strengthen relationships with staff and physicians. Why are these steps important?

References

American Medical Group Association and RSM McGladrey. 2004. *2004 Medical Group Compensation & Financial Survey*. Alexandria, VA: American Medical Group Association.

Collins, J. 2001. *Good to Great*. New York: HarperCollins.

Cooper, R. A., T. E. Getzen, and P. Laud. 2003. "Economic Expansion Is a Major Determinant of Physician Supply and Utilization." *Health Services Research* 38 (2): 675–96.

Council on Graduate Medical Education. 2000. Update on the Physician Workforce. In *U.S. Department of Health and Human Services Health Resources and Services Administration Resource Paper Compendium*. Washington, D.C.: U.S. Government Printing Office.

Donabedian, A. 1966 "Evaluating the Quality of Medical Care." *Milbank Memorial Fund Quarterly* 44: 166–206.

Lyons, T. F., and T. J. Callahan. 1996. "A Third Role in Performance Appraisal: A Suggestion from the Medical Care Quality Appraisal Systems." *Public Personnel Management* 25 (2): 133–40.

Medical Group Management Association. 2004. *MGMA Physician Compensation and Production Survey: 2004 Report Based on 2003 Data*. Englewood, CO: Medical Group Management Association.

Press-Ganey and Associates. 2005. "Press Ganey." [Online information; retrieved 2/17/05]. www.pressganey.com/.

Simmons, H. J., and J. M. Harris. 2004. "Community Based Physician Need Planning Methodologies Evolve." *Health Care Strategic Management* 22 (12): 1, 14–19.

Solucient, LLC. 2003. *Physician Community Requirements in the 21st Century: The 2003 Physicians to Population Ratios*. Evanston, IL: Solucient, LLC.

Weiner, J. P. 2004. "Prepaid Group Practice Staffing and U.S. Physician Supply: Lessons for Workforce Policy." [Online information; retrieved 2/17/05.] http://content.healthaffairs.org/cgi/gca?allch=&SEARCHID=110866674 9308_2737&AUTHOR1=weiner&JOURNALCODE=&FIRSTIN-DEX=0&hits=10&RESULTFORMAT=&gca=healthaff%3Bhlthaff.w4.43v1.

Woodcock, E. 2003. *Mastering Patient Flow: More Ideas to Increase Efficiency and Earnings*. Englewood, CO: Medical Group Management Association.

INFORMATION SYSTEMS

Rosemarie Nelson

Learning Objectives

This chapter will enable the reader to:

- identify methods to develop a needs assessment tool with practice management system features and functions to meet specific practice operational objectives;
- recognize ways in which technology training and ongoing support for staff can facilitate more effective operational processes in the clinical environment;
- identify the technology components and develop a strategy for information system technology that will result in practice growth while improving physician-patient relationships at a reasonable maintenance cost to the practice; and
- summarize an approach to speed the medical practice, including staff and patients, down the information highway to better medical recording keeping.

Chapter Purpose

This chapter outlines the critical issues in an information systems strategy for a practice, including practice management systems and electronic medical record (EMR) systems. Information systems and information management are keys to the organization and its development. Information technology can be compared to the body's central nervous system, carrying messages back and forth between providers, administrators, and the members performing tasks and services. Methods for conducting information needs assessment are described along with ways for prioritizing needs. Information systems training and support are critical components of success, for example, in database management and network security. The history and use of EMRs are traced. Current EMR systems are described, and ways in which small group practices can use them are proposed. How the EMR of the future can be used to improve both the process and outcome of medical care is explored. Barriers to the development of the EMR are defined, and ways to overcome them are suggested.

Case in Point

An administrator new to a 15-physician group practice identified a significant weakness in the group's information management capabilities. The administrator determined the best approach would be an assessment of the group's needs, prioritized for a system selection project. Because some of the group's physicians had expressed a desire to acquire an EMR, they defined the scope of the system search project to include standard practice management needs (appointment scheduling, billing and collections, and financial reporting) as well as clinical record-keeping functions expected to be found in an EMR.

Suddenly the president of the clinic appeared in the administrative offices. He said a number of physicians were objecting to the EMR because they believed its use would require them to change the way they practiced medicine. What can the administrator do to address the physicians' concerns and move the system selection project forward?

Background

Information technology (IT) appeared in physician practices in the 1980s with the adoption of early practice management systems for billing and collections. As practices realized cost savings with automating business processes, computerized patient appointment scheduling was next in the progression along the technology continuum. The personal computer (PC) brought efficiencies to the transcription process. As medical practices computerized other business functions, such as accounts payable, payroll processing, and inventory maintenance, the demand for sophisticated business reporting and clinical automation increased. Hospitals, laboratories, and ancillary testing centers initiated connectivity services for physicians to access patients' clinical information.

Increasingly sophisticated IT needs require a strategic and systematic approach to system acquisition and implementation in medical practices. The interconnectedness and layers of functionality affecting a single medical practice are shown in Figure 7.1.

Information System Implementation

Goals and Objectives

The first step in determining IT needs is the definition of the medical practice's goals and objectives. Strategic planning determines where the medical practice is going over the next three to five years. The IT plan must be developed within the context of the medical practice's strategic goals and objectives.

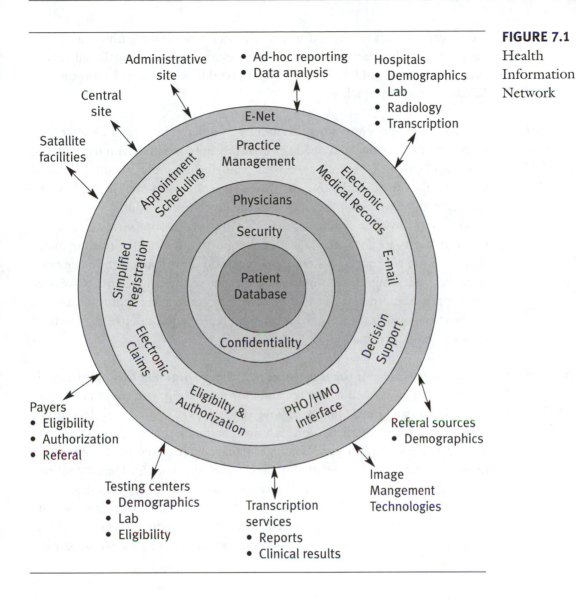

FIGURE 7.1
Health Information Network

A data strategy identifies the group's plans to build a data infrastructure and the use of data standards. The migration and implementation strategy describes the sequencing of projects, including infrastructure and application acquisition, and implementation and organizational change.

Process and Needs Assessment

With the vision and mission defined by the strategic plan, the medical practice can perform a process assessment. The practice may determine through an assessment that operations can be enhanced by modified processes. A process assessment completed prior to a system implementation provides the opportunity to match a vendor offering to the strategic goals and objectives as defined in the planning phase. A workflow analysis that focuses on how an individual's work is sequenced and how work is transferred within the organization is a preliminary task in process redesign. An operational analysis addresses the "why" and "what for" behind workflow and aims to improve efficiencies as well as quality.

Interdisciplinary, Interdepartmental Teams

A process and needs assessment should be completed by interdisciplinary, interdepartmental teams of individuals involved and intimately familiar with the workflow and processes. A successful team includes the nursing, medical records, front-desk, and business office departments as well as a physician representative. An initial orientation to the capabilities, including efficiencies as well as quality improvements, that IT can provide is necessary to prepare the team for its assignment. Educational opportunities include reading materials, web site references, system demonstration downloads, vendor demonstrations, and seminars. A single management team, consultant, or vendor can support the process, but the effort will be more successful if performed by those responsible for change and system implementation, like the interdisciplinary project team.

Chart Current and Desired Workflow

During the assessment the team must create an environment within the medical practice that is open to change and looking for opportunities to eliminate redundancies and streamline workflow. One method that effectively engages participants in change discussions is a flowchart of a current process and the desired process or ideal state. Change management is key to the successful implementation of IT. The total quality management (TQM) and continuous quality improvement (CQI) techniques have been incorporated by many industries, including healthcare, in successfully modifying operations. Creating new revenue opportunities (see Appendix 7.1), reducing costs, and improving patient service and quality of care are results of process assessment projects.

Inventory Current Capabilities

An early step in the needs identification process is to inventory current capabilities. It is not a given that all systems are created equal. By establishing the baseline or minimum set of requirements of those features and functions the group already enjoys, the assessment team can build the functional capabilities that may be missing; inventory the applications that already exist (e.g., transcription systems, lab resulting reporting, Internet availability for patient education materials); review all reports used daily, weekly, and monthly to determine the extent of current use as well as information missing or in demand; and document by user the applications—and their features and functions—used on a daily, weekly, and monthly basis that will further define the minimum needs for subsequent technology solutions.

Identifying needs often begins by surveying users. Observation of operations and validation of process flowcharts provide a secondary checkpoint in the needs assessment phase. An initial introduction to IT capabilities is helpful to users who may have limited exposure to systems and therefore may not identify needs to the depth and breadth with which a system can meet them.

For example, if administration is not aware that by using billing and appointment data the medical practice could recall patients based on chronic diagnoses and prior dates of service for specific procedures, that department may not identify revenue-generating recall opportunities as a function of the practice management systems. Another example is the nurse who does not realize that a computerized physician order entry (CPOE) system would provide the status of tests without the need to telephone the testing centers and include CPOE as a core feature of the electronic medical record (EMR).

Surveys can be approached many ways (see Appendix 7.2). Open-ended questions such as, "What information do you need to access in the EMR?" are best suited to the visionaries who are actively engaged in the process. Providing insight to potential process improvements with survey questions such as, "Could clinical message routing linked to e-mail be effectively integrated into your workflow?" will help those who claim to be non-technical understand the scope of change a new information system will bring.

An IT assessment must ask how the system supports patient flow, appointment scheduling, cash collections, and data queries. A sample practice management system needs assessment that allows users to apply a weighting factor to each feature and function is provided in Appendix 7.3. The same checklist can be subsequently used in scoring vendor demonstrations.

Effective Technology Training and Disbursement

One key factor in successful system implementation is a support infrastructure for staff. A technology training plan for clinical and administrative staff along with continual process redesign by an interdisciplinary, interdepartmental team bring improvements to daily operations. This must include an understanding of the language and definitions used in information systems (see Appendix 7.4).

For example, nursing staff skilled in PC applications can more readily adopt the use of a PC network and file management tool to access transcribed office notes to support patient telephone triage. An electronic access point to dictated reports and lab results reduces the need to pull charts and eliminates delays for patients, both resulting in lower overhead costs and improved service. Another example of effective technology training and disbursement is the decentralization of appointment scheduling. Technology-trained nurses can schedule follow-up appointments at the point of care rather than pushing the task to a checkout function where the authority to work appointments into a calendar at capacity is lacking.

System and Vendor Selection

Practice management and EMR systems are typically based in three primary architectures: mainframe, client-server, and Web based.

Many legacy systems are mainframe systems, the primary configuration for the medical environment in the early 1980s. The mainframe is a single central computer that performs all processing and storage functions accessed by dumb terminals (workstations with no processing capabilities of their own). UNIX is one operating system that supports the central processor configuration.

The client-server environment was the next phase of technology offered to medical practices. Several computers (servers) perform much of the processing and resource-intensive tasks (building data queries, processing electronic claims, producing patient statements, and so on), while the clients (PC workstations) access the servers to capture and view data. The clients may also process minor transactions, such as a BMI calculation from the entry of a patient's vital statistics.

The most current architecture is Web based and allows workstations running Web browsers to interact with the system for data capture and display.

Many of the current vendor offerings in the marketplace use a mixture of architectures, with the various components advantageously based on the desired functionality. For example, a client-server system may provide remote access via a Web-based interface for physicians or for patients interacting with limited components of their electronic health records (EHRs). A secure Internet connection to the medical practice EHR might allow patients to submit updates to their medications via a chart similar to that shown in Table 7.1. The patient's Web-based interface would become a component of the medical practice's client-server EMR.

The process and needs assessment becomes one of the tools to evaluate the products and vendors offering technology solutions to meet the medical practice's strategic plan. Although features and functions are high-profile elements of the system selection, identifying a vendor that provides services to match the group's culture and orientation is a significant factor in the ultimate success of the implementation. IT skills are often acquired via direct experience, and Table 7.2 explores some potential experiences every group must examine as it selects the best-fit product and vendor. Vendor relationship management is critical to successful EMR implementation.

Computerized patient records have been in the marketplace since the 1980s. EMRs have been developed by practice management systems companies as they recognized the next phase of their market's needs. Start-up companies also began to deliver EMRs as the increasing capabilities of IT offered

Prescriptions						
Name of medicine	Dose Total (mg)	How many times per day?	When do you take it? (Morning and night? After meals?)	Who prescribed it for you? (Physician's last name)	Why do you take it?	Do you have any side-effects? (Describe them)
Over-the-Counter Medications, Herbal Remedies, Vitamins						

TABLE 7.1

Medication Chart Sample

SOURCE: Physicians Practice, Inc. 2002.

development tools, graphical user interface (Windows), and PCs with powerful processing, memory, and storage.

Early adopters found the initial product offerings limited in clinical orientation. To overcome this barrier vendors moved to acquire experience with practical applications to derive specialty-specific data entry structure and clinical protocols. As products evolved the market began to differentiate the various offerings, and Table 7.3 defines some of the industry's acronyms.

Obstacles to Electronic Medical Record (EMR) Implementation

For more than a decade EMR adoption rates stagnated at 5 to 10 percent of medical practices. Lack of capital is most frequently cited as the reason medical groups have not implemented EMRs and other clinically focused

TABLE 7.2 Vendor Management	Steps a Medical Practice Should Take to Manage Technology Vendors Effectively	What to Ask the Potential Vendor Partner
	Appreciate the value of various technology investments and their cost:benefit ratio	What are the equipment requirements? Does the application require the latest gadget and a state-of-the-art PC replaced every year?
	Understand that systems are dynamic and need to be constantly aligned with changing conditions	How do you approach downtime, when no problems or questions are coming in, and how do you stay engaged with customers to anticipate needs and application of technology solutions?
	Be dedicated to training all staff to keep technology and operations aligned	What is your approach to disseminating technology on an ongoing basis? How do you manage that process?
	Employ a multidisciplinary approach to strategic information systems and IT decision making	How do you include nontechnical staff in a technical process to achieve buy-in and enthusiasm for the adoption of new technology?
	Maintain clear accountability for the multitude of tasks and activities involved in systems and technology management	How do you manage urgent requests while maintaining progress on longer-term projects?

technology, according to data compiled by the Medical Group Management Association (MGMA) and released in 2004.

Groups that have not implemented an EMR system cited lack of capital resources as the number-one reason (cited by 25 percent); followed by lack of physician support (15 percent); insufficient time to select, contract for, install, and implement a system (10 percent); insufficient return on investment (9 percent); and inability to easily input historical medical record data into an the system (8 percent). Other reasons cited included an inability to integrate the EMR with practice billing and claims submission systems, lack of standards, lack of support from practice administrators, and security concerns.

One way to overcome some of these obstacles is to adopt an incremental approach to EMR implementation. Online access to transcribed office notes will improve responsiveness to telephone triage and improve the quality of care provided to patients. To gain access to dictated reports from any PC on the office network, create folders for each provider on the network and electronically file each transcribed report using a standard naming convention such as LastnameFirstnameYYYYMMDD-OV. Give triage nurses access to the providers' file folders and train all staff in how to find a patient file.

Electronic test results reports will also enhance quality of care and reduce costs of operations by eliminating chart pulls to respond to patient requests for test results. Add a fax server to the medical practice computer network and receive results reports electronically. Use the same standard file-naming convention (LastnameFirstnameYYYYMMDD-lab), and electronically file results in the same folder with transcription. Another method to electronically access these documents is by acquiring and implementing a document management system.

Interactive Web services to allow patients to request prescription reissues will improve the practice's refill process (Niedzwiecki et al. 2000). An electronic prescription management system for each patient can improve outcomes through the proactive management of medications for chronic disease states, which allows the practice to recall the patient at appropriate follow-up intervals.

EMR adoption rates began to increase in late 2004. The economic benefits are faster communications, less paper, and fewer chart pulls. The practice will experience fewer mistakes and less uncompensated work and see more patients more efficiently.

The EMR market continues to evolve with vendor mergers and acquisitions. Software applications and systems are absorbed and integrated within

		TABLE 7.3
Computerized Patient Record (CPR)	Computer-stored record of health information about one person linked by a personal identifier (longitudinal record)	Healthcare IT Acronyms
Electronic Patient Record/ Electronic Health Record (EPR/EHR)	Collective vision of many systems and components (derived from relevant patient information)	
Electronic Medical Record (EMR)	Interoperability between incompatible, disparate systems (stepping stone toward EPR)	
Digital Medical Record (DMR)	Vision of Web-based tool (functionality of EMR or EPR)	
Continuity of Care Record (CCR)	Technology neutral and intended to foster and improve continuity of patient care and ensure at least a minimum level of quality when a patient is referred, transferred, or otherwise goes to another provider setting	

products. Technology changes approximately every 18 months. Monitoring change positions an organization to plan for incorporating new developments into its strategic vision.

Summary

This chapter reviews methods for the development of a needs assessment tool that has practice management system features and functions that meet specific practice operational objectives. It emphasizes the need for technology training and continuous staff support for more effective operational processes. The technology components and strategies for information system technology implementation for practice growth and effectiveness and efficiency improvement are described. The utility of the EMR is considered, and various methods to develop automated approaches to the information highway, especially for small practices, are described. Barriers to that development are also defined with approaches for breaking them down.

Discussion Questions

1. What are the early steps in planning an information system acquisition?
2. How can you create an environment in which technology is successfully exploited?
3. What technology could you employ to engage patients in their medical record keeping?
4. Describe how IT supports the medical practice's daily operations and strategic vision.

References

Medical Group Management Association. 2004. "Research Connexion." [Online information; retrieved 2/21/05.] www.mgma.com/research/emr.cfm.

Niedzwiecki, P., S. L. Priest, V. C. Pivnicny, and B. C. Ruffino. 2000. "Leveraging HIPAA to Support Consumer Empowerment." *Journal of Healthcare Information Management* 14 (4): 95–104.

APPENDIX 7.1 RETURN ON INVESTMENT (ROI) CALCULATION WORKSHEET

Part 1: Direct Equipment Cost

_____ Purchase Price

+ _____Finance Costs

+ _____Facility Modifications

= _____Direct Equipment Cost

_____ Years for Payback

_____ Annual Utilization

Divide Direct Equipment Cost by Years for Payback and Utilization

_____ Direct Equipment Cost per Procedure

Part 2: Supply and Utility Cost

_____ Annual Supply Cost

+ _____Annual Utility Costs

= _____Annual Supply and Utility Cost

_____ Annual Utilization

Divide Annual Supply and Utility Cost by Utilization

_____ Supply and Utility Cost per Procedure

Part 3: Direct Labor Cost

Step 1—Estimate Staff Labor Costs

_____ Average Salary per Full-time Equivalent (FTE)

+ _____Benefits

= _____Labor Cost per FTE

Step 2—Estimate Staff Time for Equipment

_____ FTE to Operate

_____ Annual Utilization

Multiply Labor Cost per FTE by FTE to Operate and Divide by Annual Utilization

_____ Labor Cost per Procedure

Part 4: Cost Savings

_____ Costs of Previous Technology or Process

+ _____Labor Costs for Positions Deleted

_____ Cost Savings per Year

_____ Annual Utilization
Divide Cost Savings by Annual Utilization
_____ Cost Savings per Procedure

Part 5: Training Costs

_____ Initial Training Costs (First Year)
_____ Time Period for Payback
Divide Initial Training Costs by Time Period for Payback
= _____ Amortized Initial Training Costs
+ _____ Annual Training Costs After First Year
= _____ Annual Training Costs
_____ Annual Utilization
Divide Cost Savings by Annual Utilization
_____ Annual Training Costs per Procedure

Part 6: Direct Revenue

_____ Revenue per Procedure

Part 7: Revenue from Increased Productivity

_____ Increased Provider Procedures (Office Visit, Surgical Procedure)
_____ Revenue per Procedure
Multiply Increased Provider Procedures by Revenue
_____ Total Revenue from Increased Productivity

_____ Direct Equipment Cost per Procedure
+ _____ Supply and Utility Cost per Procedure
+ _____ Labor Cost per Procedure
− _____ Cost Savings per Procedure
− _____ Annual Training Costs per Procedure
+ _____ Revenue per Procedure
= _____ Net Revenue per Procedure
Multiply by Utilization
= _____ Annual Net Revenue
+ _____ Total Revenue from Increased Productivity
= _____ Annual Revenue to Practice

SOURCE: Gans, D. N., director, Practice Management Resources, MGMA. 2004.

APPENDIX 7.2 ELECTRONIC MEDICAL RECORD (EMR) CHECKLIST

Thinking about implementing an EMR in your practice? Dublin Primary Care in Colorado Springs, Colorado, successfully introduced the technology to its staff and patients. Debbie Milburn, CMPE, operations manager and an MGMA member, assisted in establishing this tool. She offers a checklist for practices to use as they take the plunge.

Decision Making
- Consider your practice's long-range planning.
  - Make your practice management, billing, and EMR decisions at the same time.
  - Is this a proper goal based on your financial status?
  - Understand the costs of paper medical records, such as printing, paper, and other hidden expenses.
  - Perform a return on investment (ROI) analysis.
- Decide as a group to implement the EMR. Take a look at the benefits:
  - Reduced staffing
  - Easier to comply with regulations
  - Transfer of information (site to site) easier and more efficient
- Take a look at the downsides:
  - Implementation of computer systems difficult
  - Practice has other projects and not enough time and resources to implement EMR
  - Cashflow not strong enough to withstand implementation
- Get all your physicians and administrators on board.
  - Hold a meeting to discuss and make everyone a part of the decision.
  - Listen to issues, comments, and suggestions.
  - Agree to implement with a positive attitude from all staff.
- Look at the EMR products available (via the Internet, exhibit halls at conferences, an so on).
  - Review the ability of products to interface with your existing practice management programs.
- Locate a local practice using an EMR and ask questions.
  - Talk to physicians.
  - Talk to administrators.
  - Ask how they use the system and how they like it.
  - What improvements do both groups recognize?
  - Did documentation improve as a result of the implementation?

- Locate a vendor that meets your price and service needs.
  — Does it provide on-site training?
  — How long is the transition between training and support?
  — What kind of warranty is offered?
- Ask for references and ask the clients to:
  — identify the positives and negatives experienced during implementation;
  — talk about the level of service provided by the vendor;
  — discuss maintenance issues (what has happened since the implementation); and
  — review their experience meshing the EMR system with other vendors' products.

Implementation
- Create a plan to include:
  — time frame (it is critical to implement as quickly as possible);
  — tasks and responsibilities;
  — mandatory training for all staff; and
  — commitment of key physicians and staff.
- Implement EMR with a vendor representative on site.
- Schedule and complete training.
- Ensure that vendor support is available.
- Assess security for both hardware and software.

Maintenance
- Make sure you incorporate service agreements in your contract.
- Know the limitations of the service contract (time available, how it is measured, and so on).

SOURCE: MGMA 2003.

APPENDIX 7.3 SAMPLE PRACTICE MANAGEMENT NEEDS ASSESSMENT

Practice Management Information Systems			
Weight Factor (1 = Nice; 2 = Need; 3 = Must Have)	Description and Rating Score (0 = Not Available; 1 = Low; 2 = Average; 3 = Good; Blank = Unknown)	System 1 Score	System 2 Score
General			
1	Online help		
3	Limits user access to specific functions		
3	Produces audit trail of transaction entries and master file updates		
Practice Operations			
2	Assigns action items and ticklers for patient accounts to users		
1	Messaging and tickles by type and date		
3	Allows batch report jobs with scheduled time, day, and frequency as specified by user		
3	Submit claims electronically with any frequency		
3	Produces patient statements weekly with cycle repetition		
3	Maintains multiple fee schedules based on payer		
Patient Appointment Scheduling			
3	Scheduling by type for providers and other resources or rooms		
3	Allocates time based on appointment type parameters as varied by provider		
2	Schedules multiple resources at one time		
2	Schedules providers across multiple locations		
3	Easily maintains provider schedule changes (bumps, cancellations)		

Practice Management Information Systems			
Weight Factor (1 = Nice; 2 = Need; 3 = Must Have)	Description and Rating Score (0 = Not Available; 1 = Low; 2 = Average; 3 = Good; Blank = Unknown)	System 1 Score	System 2 Score
3	Allows mini-admit or quick registration of patients for scheduling		
3	Produces reports, encounter slips, and requisitions from schedule by provider or resource		
2	Produces report of patients with appointments but no charges		
1	Allows tracking of patient arrival, room, and exit status		
Patient Account Management			
3	Maintains patient and insurance balances		
3	Creates recall by patient, procedure, or mass query (e.g., all women over 40 with no mammogram history)		
1	Tracks referral source		
2	Maintains patient-preferred pharmacy		
1	Permits maintenance of family accounts with multiple patients linked to one guarantor		
3	Permits at least three insurance sources per patient		
1	Some user-defined fields and free-form notes		
2	Maintain insurance authorization and referral information, including codes, effective dates, procedures, and diagnoses		
1	Maintains copayment amounts		
3	Ease of use for navigation through functions		
3	Quick entry of patient registration information		
3	Checkout function accepts payment, schedules appointments, and prints receipt or invoice with new appointment date and time scheduled		
3	Daily operator balance report for audit trail and daily reconciliation		

Practice Management Information Systems			
Weight Factor (1 = Nice; 2 = Need; 3 = Must Have)	Description and Rating Score (0 = Not Available; 1 = Low; 2 = Average; 3 = Good; Blank = Unknown)	System 1 Score	System 2 Score
3	Transactions tagged with date, time, and operator		
Payments			
1	Alerts user to insurance payments that vary from profile stored in system		
3	Calculates adjustments and write-offs based on allowed amounts (e.g., Medicare)		
3	Automatic secondary or tertiary bill generated on payment		
3	Accepts electronic remittance		
3	Line-item posting with full history of all postings		
Collections			
3	Produces reports by exception criteria (over X dollars and over X days old) stratified by balance		
3	Provides insurance analysis reporting		
1	Payment plan function		
1	Includes letter writing for bad debt account sequenced after patient statements		
3	Exports file format for electronic transfer to collection services		
3	Reports by provider, location, department, or specialty		
Management Reports			
3	Analyzes by provider, zip code, insurance, location, procedure, diagnosis, modifier, and combinations		
3	Amount of payment and adjustments by insurance, provider, or location		
1	Mailing labels for individuals, families, and insurance companies		
3	Insurance allowable and payment versus profile maintained		
	Total		

APPENDIX 7.4 LANGUAGE AND DEFINITIONS USED IN INFORMATION SYSTEMS

Computer System Infrastructure

Input	PC (desktop, notebook, tablet); dumb terminal; personal digital assistant (PDA); electronic data interchange (EDI); digital fax; voice
Output	Display devices (PC, dumb terminal, PDA); EDI; digital fax; printer
Network and Communications; Application Processing and Data Storage	Mainframe; client-server; Web-based

Network Configuration

Local Area Network (LAN)	Group of computers connected within a relatively small geographic area, generally through dedicated cable
Wireless LAN (WLAN)	Wireless devices that connects to a LAN via radio waves
Wide Area Network (WAN)	Group of computers that connect across larger geographic distances via telephone or cable services
Virtual Private Network (VPN)	A WAN that uses a private tunnel through the Internet rather than privately owned cable or leased lines
Internet Service Provider (ISP)	Organization providing leased connectivity to the Internet

Physical Topology

Bus	Simple backbone device connectivity

Star	Central hub acts as traffic cop
Ring	Computers connected via cable arranged in a ring, computer to computer

Logical Topology

Token Ring	Ring physical topology with a token that passes computer to computer to ensure that only one computer transmits data at a time
Ethernet	Most popular; uses a pause to ensure that data do not collide; network-specific cables (e.g., 10Base2, 10Base5, 10BaseT)
Asynchronous Transfer Mode (ATM)	One of the newest topologies; carries both voice and data over network wire or fiber

Network Components

Network Operating System (NOS)	Family of programs that run the ne worked computers; most common are Windows 2000, Windows NT, and UNIX
Network Interface Card (NIC)	LAN adapters, wireless access cards; create packages of data that enhance strength of low-powered digital signals to enable packages to travel through a transmission medium
Hub	Central location where cables on network come together
Bridge	Enables computers on separate networks or parts of a network to exchange information
Routers	Connectors that link different networks
Switch	May replace bridge-router combination

Network Protocols	Rules for Sending and Receiving Data Across a Network
Transmission Control Protocol (TCP)	Used to transfer information between two devices on a network
Internet Protocol (IP)	Responsible for addressing information
TCP/IP	Collection of protocols
File Transfer Protocol (FTP)	Used to transfer documents between different types of computers
Hypertext Transfer Protocol (HTTP)	Used to transfer information from Web servers to Web browsers

BUSINESS AND CLINICAL OPERATIONS

Rosemarie Nelson

Learning Objectives

This chapter will enable the reader to:

- identify best practices in patient flow and the provision of services;
- describe methods to evaluate, measure, and monitor patient satisfaction and quality activities within medical practice operations;
- recognize ways in which clinical services can be monitored in single- and multispecialty group settings;
- summarize an approach to evaluate the business potential of offering ancillary services within the scope of the practice; and
- discuss the use of nonphysician providers in the medical practice setting.

Chapter Purpose

This chapter identifies business and clinical operations that contribute to the efficiencies of a medical practice at the highest level of satisfaction for providers, employees, and patients. Patient flow and the provision of services in an efficient and effective manner are critical. This is a function of how well staff are trained and organized along with the physical layout of the facilities where the services are provided. Functionality should be the key performance measure. Quality and patient satisfaction and the methods for measuring these key factors are described from both process and outcome perspectives. A myriad of clinical services can be provided by the organization, and the use and misuse of ancillary and clinical support services are described. The use of nonphysician providers is also considered.

Case in Point

The physicians of a mid-sized medical practice approached the administrator with a strong conviction that the group absolutely had to cut back on overhead and expand service offerings because personal income had been decreasing. The administrator recommended to the physicians that they undertake an overall operational assessment and survey their staff and patients to learn where opportunities for efficiencies could be gained and identify services in demand by patients.

One of the physicians complained that this was just a stall. He discussed the matter with the president, who then scheduled a meeting with the administrator. How can the administrator approach this discussion of assessing the efficient delivery of current services?

Practice Operations

Successful medical practice operations are based on strategic business planning (see Chapter 4), leadership (see Chapter 2), and teamwork. A key to the process of business planning is monitoring the plan, an annual process described in Chapter 4. Based on prioritized goals and objectives the medical practice can determine operational parameters to benchmark and monitor in order to measure the success rate of operational change to meet those goals and objectives. Training and motivating staff, as outlined in Chapter 6, are the essential activities for the development of an effective team. The operations manager must build a team that can support the billable provider to maximize productivity and meet the organization's operational goals. Benchmarking, the continual process of measuring and comparing key work process indicators, demonstrates how to improve performance and profitability in practice operations.

Patient Flow and the Provision of Services

Practice operations begin with workflow design in the delivery of services to patients. The optimal design for patient flow, whether in the office or over the telephone, is the difference between the successful practice and the practice teetering on insolvency.

Redesign of Telephone Flow

The initial point of contact for most patients is the telephone. Recognizing that approximately 100 phone calls are received daily for a provider with a base of 1,500 to 2,500 active patients, skilled staff members supporting telephone flow are essential to smooth operational flow.

Track Incoming Calls   To effectively serve patients and perform efficiently an initial benchmark of incoming calls is a place to begin the redesign of telephone flow. Track incoming calls (see Table 8.1 for a sample call log) for a period of two to four weeks to determine the reason for the calls.

Call Log: Root Cause Analysis				
Date	Staff initials	Date of last appointment? (Ask or look up)	Repeat?	Reason for call (Summary)

TABLE 8.1
Sample Call Log

Summarize and Analyze Tracked Calls

Summarize the tracked calls by (1) timing post-appointment and (2) subject matter. Typically 30 to 40 percent of calls are from patients who have been seen in the prior two weeks. Are those calls that could be prevented by anticipating the patients' needs at the time of the appointment and integrating them into the exam? Patient calls regarding prescription refills indicate opportunities to query patients at the time of their exam regarding medication management. Incoming calls to ask for test results signal that expectations have not been set appropriately.

Applying a change in process and tracking calls three months postintervention is a good method to measure the effectiveness of the operational change. For example, Figure 8.1 demonstrates an alternative method to report lab results to patients via secure telephone and Web site access.

Chart Staff and Patient Contact

Flowchart each point of staff contact in the patient office and telephone encounter to identify potential work redesign. By reengineering patient flow processes to minimize staff members' contact with patients and eliminate rework, operations can be streamlined and patient satisfaction will improve. For example, collecting the patient's copayment responsibility during the check-in process eliminates the need for the patient to present at a checkout station after the appointment.

Survey Patient Satisfaction

Simple surveys of patients can highlight areas for operational improvement. A survey like the sample shown in Table 8.2, if introduced to the patient at check-in or checkout, can be used before and after workflow modification has been undertaken.

FIGURE 8.1
Lab Results
Delivery

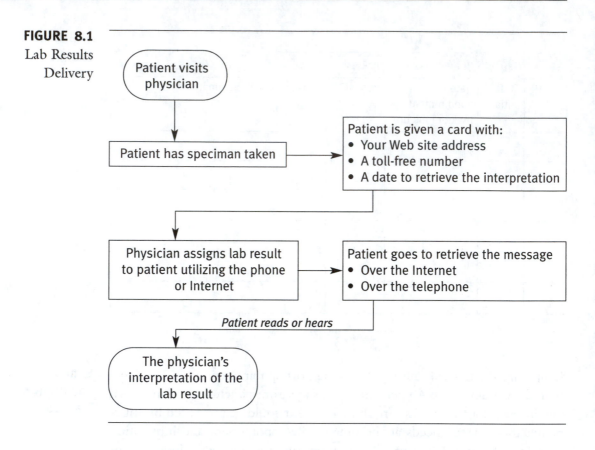

More sophisticated methods such as patient focus groups and extensive telephone survey instruments are other tools medical practices employ to monitor their performance. Engaging external expertise to develop and implement the survey tools is an objective measure that is most beneficial when repeated at routine intervals to determine the success rate of interventions applied as a result of survey findings.

Efficient Appointment Scheduling

Effective patient flow in the office is a result of efficient appointment scheduling. To maintain timely service to patients and optimal provider productivity better-performing practices automate patient appointment reminders. Automated reminder systems typically interface with practice management systems as demonstrated in Figure 8.2. The practice management systems in which the patient contact information and appointments are maintained, is queried to develop a subset of patients scheduled for appointments two to three days in the future. This resulting subset is transferred to the automated appointment reminder application, which subsequently contacts the patients using the telephone numbers stored in the practice management system to deliver reminder messages to the patients. Automation of the workflow to remind patients of their appointments is an efficient and economical way to reduce the rate of patients who miss their appointments.

Physical Facility Efficiency

The physical facility can contribute to effective patient flow and provider productivity or constrain the operation from efficiently offering specific services. A pod of exam rooms and an alcove for provider messaging and charting can save footsteps and time, allowing the provider to see an additional one or two patients each day. Small work units maximize communication and visibility and minimize distances between tasks.

How the provider's time is spent during the encounter should be observed to ensure that exam rooms are properly stocked with supplies so providers do not have to leave the exam room during the encounter. Standardized exam rooms, with supplies and patient educational material always stored in the same drawer or cabinet, add flexibility by allowing providers to use the rooms interchangeably. This can increase throughput and reduce the constraint of too few exam rooms.

The provider messaging and charting alcove becomes a virtual fourth exam room where the provider can return messages, respond to nurse inquiries, review incoming test results and correspondence, and complete patient documentation. A line-of-sight view of the exam room pod from the nursing station facilitates efficient flow. If the facility design does not permit a straight line of sight, technology can be used to support the operation

TABLE 8.1
Sample Call Log

	Very Satisfied	Acceptable	Dissatisfied
How long you waited to get an appointment			
Getting through to the office by phone			
Length of time waiting at the office			
Time spent with your provider			
Technical skills (thoroughness, carefulness, competence) of your provider			
Personal manner (courtesy, respect, sensitivity, friendliness) of your provider			
This visit overall			

Comments:

FIGURE 8.2
Appointment
Reminder
Application

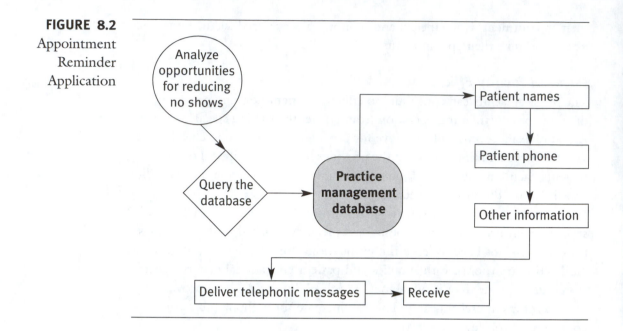

through instant messaging between staff and clinicians or by directing forms to print to workstations as signals of patient arrivals or order requests.

Adequate Patient Service Training for Staff

Staff members supporting the medical group's operations require patient service training in addition to their required duties to perform at high levels in their roles. In the competitive healthcare environment customer service differentiates one medical practice from another in a community. Service standards and operational indicators are measures of success. The nine elements of service, as reported by Delio in *The Perfect Practice for an Efficient Physician* (1999), are:

- **Efficacy**: Did the service achieve the desired outcome?
- **Appropriateness**: Is the service appropriate under the circumstances?
- **Availability**: Is the service available to the patient?
- **Timeliness**: Is the service performed in a timely manner that meets the patient's expectation?
- **Effectiveness**: Is the service completed in a beneficial manner?
- **Continuity**: Is there consideration as to how the next steps will be performed?
- **Safety**: Is the environment safe for the patient?
- **Efficiency**: Is there a relationship between the care and resources needed?
- **Respect and caring**: Is the patient involved, and is confidentiality ensured?

Service begins with a well-organized and trained staff. Better-performing practices develop orientation schedules for all individuals new to the practice. Orient clinical staff, nurses, and providers to all aspects of the practice to achieve a working team with respect and appreciation for operational processes and procedures. The revenue cycle—from scheduling an appointment for a new patient through posting the final payment against that encounter—should be clearly understood by all members of the medical practice. The lowest level of performance by any employee that is allowed to continue without corrective action becomes the highest level of performance that can be required of any other employee in a similar position with the group. Training and staff development are ongoing processes essential to reaching operational excellence.

Measures to Monitor Performance

Operational Indicators

A medical practice must identify measures to monitor performance and opportunities for improvement. Operational indicators can be extracted from the practice's practice management system and benchmarked against industry standards such as those recommended by the Medical Group Management Association (Schryver 2002). Benchmarks can be compared against practices that are similar in specialty, size, organization, and geographic region. Better-performing practices analyze trends and patterns and extrapolate meaningful information from practice utilization data. Sample metrics that can be measured on a daily or monthly basis and trended over a rolling period or reported month to month and year to year are:

- Support staff full-time equivalent (FTE) per provider and payroll hours
- Accounts receivable over 120 days old and write-offs
- Productivity per provider (annual visits, procedures, relative value units, clinic hours)
- Payer mix
- Cash collected
- Charge lag time
- Patient visit cycle time with specific wait times within the cycle (e.g., answer phone, time to appointment, reception, exam room, referral, results)
- No-show rates
- Denial rates by payer and reason
- Patient call-backs
- On-call patient responses
- Total medical revenue after operating cost per FTE physician

- Total operating cost as percentage of total medical revenue
- Triage calls and minutes on call
- Percentage of patients with complete and accurate registration collected at time of scheduling the next available appointment

Clinical Indicators

Clinical indicators of quality of care may appear more difficult to measure when considering traditional methods such as evaluating medical chart documentation. Previsit preparation as well as retrospective examination of clinical performance will position a medical practice to meet payer standards, which is critical in contract reimbursement negotiations. Preparation for the visit begins with a preview of the chart using a specialty-specific tool similar to the example in Table 8.3.

Retrospective review of clinical activities can present measurable data. According to a RAND Health Report published in the *New England Journal of Medicine* (McGlynn et al. 2003), patients receive roughly 55 percent of the recommended care for preventive (e.g., cancer screening), acute (e.g., ear infection), and chronic (e.g., diabetes) needs. The Centers for Disease Control reports from 1995 through 1997 provided similar findings: Only 52 percent of adults over age 65 received an annual influenza vaccine, and only 67 percent of women over age 18 had a Pap smear in the prior three years.

Finite Measures of Clinical Activities

Finite measures of clinical activities can be evaluated and monitored routinely even without benefit of an EMR by virtually all practices. Using the practice management system the medical practice can report services by current procedural terminology (CPT) code, date of service, patient demographics (gender, age, geographic location), and diagnosis using International Classification of Disease (ICD) codes. A simple query of the practice management system can readily identify all patients due for a Pap smear or overdue for immunizations.

Whether driven by pay-for-performance standards or a group practice's strategic vision, clinical protocols can be monitored and reported effectively with billing data from the practice management system. Tracking referrals ordered for patients through the system provides another measure of clinical services on a provider level.

Referral Tracking and Management

Referral tracking and management is a barometer of revenue potential for both single- and multispecialty groups. For example, if a primary care provider in a practice has a disproportionate volume of patient referrals to otolaryngologists, that may indicate an opportunity for additional continuing medical education in that area. Enhancing the provider's knowledge and skill

TABLE 8.3
Patient Chart
Prep Tool

Test	Date	Action Required
CBC		
EKG		
Urinalysis		
Mammogram		
Cholesterol, triglycerides, LDL, HDL		
Immunizations		

set may result in keeping patients in the practice for some services—rather than referring the patient out—and therefore increasing the revenue to the practice.

However, the potential to misuse the provision of additional services does exist. A provider who seeks out and obtains training on a specific procedure, such as sigmoidoscopy, may order screening tests inappropriately in an attempt to take advantage of the additional revenue the procedure's reimbursement provides to the practice.

Additional Services Analysis

Community Need

Medical groups' interests keep pace as new opportunities arise; current areas include esthetic procedures, wound care, obesity treatment, sleep disorder treatment, infusion treatment, products for sale (e.g., vitamins), screening procedures, rehabilitation and therapy, and surgery centers or specialty hospitals. Participation in clinical studies can benefit the practice and its patients. National firms offer franchise-like services including set-up and staffing for new services. A gap analysis identifies service lines that match community needs. A strengths, weaknesses, opportunities, and threats analysis is one input to the development of a business plan for ancillary revenue opportunities.

Financial Assessment

The business plan, as outlined in Chapter 4, addresses the strategic issues for the practice's growth and revenue diversification. During the planning process options are prioritized for selection and implementation. Each option must be analyzed from a financial, legal, and operational perspective. Is the new service clinically appropriate and medically necessary as well as consistent with the values and business sense of the practice? The financial assessment answers the questions of patient demand, payers and reimbursement, and expenses to start and maintain the service. Evaluation of legal feasibility and the business model for development may require expertise outside the practice. Political considerations within the community may carry more weight in the final determination.

Use of Nonphysician Providers

The use of nonphysician providers can increase the revenue generated within medical practices directly or indirectly. In some practices a nonphysician provider (e.g., nurse practitioner) will develop a base of patients that increases the active patient base for the practice. In other practices the nonphysician provider (e.g., physician assistant) extends the physician's productivity by sharing the care of hospital inpatients to assist with history and physicals for new admissions and for patient rounding and discharges. Nonphysician providers often provide postoperative care and handle same-day acute visits that cannot be scheduled on the physician's calendar immediately.

Summary

Medical practices operate in a complicated environment regulated by government and payer organizations; at the same time they are evaluated by patients every day. Groups that perform self-assessments and monitor operational performance in the quest to continuously improve efficiencies and exceed patient expectations are better performers year after year. Well-trained, organized staff in an effective facility with satisfied providers will contribute to a practice dedicated to meeting its mission and serving its patients.

Discussion Questions

1. What are the key operational indicators necessary to manage effective service to patients?
2. What information should be extracted from the practice management system to determine potential new services to incorporate into the medical practice?
3. What are some of the changes a practice can make to reduce incoming patient telephone volume?
4. How would you evaluate patient satisfaction regarding your medical practice operations?
5. What role can nonphysician providers play in the group practice setting?

References

Delio, S. A. 1999. *The Perfect Practice for an Efficient Physician*. Englewood, CO: Medical Group Management Association.

McGlynn, E. A., S. M. Asch, J. Adams, J. Keesey, J. Hicks, A. DeCristofaro, and E. A. Kerr. 2003. "The Quality of Health Care Delivered to Adults in the United States." *New England Journal of Medicine* 348 (26): 2635–45.

Schryver, D. L. (Ed.). 2002. *Assessment Manual for Medical Groups*. Englewood, CO: Medical Group Management Association.

QUALITY ASSESSMENT, RISK EVALUATION, AND MANAGED CARE

Frederick J. Wenzel

Learning Objectives

This chapter will enable the reader to:

- understand the need for and value of quality assessment;
- apply methods to evaluate quality;
- understand the difference between process and outcome methodologies;
- understand the complexity of quality evaluation;
- recognize the need to evaluate risk in the organization;
- understand the history and development of managed care organizations; and
- evaluate the impact of managed care on the healthcare system.

Chapter Purpose

This chapter considers quality assessment and improvement from a variety of perspectives. First is differentiating the professional's point of view from that of the patient. A discussion of the various methods of evaluating quality, emphasizing the differences between outcome and process assessment, follows. A sophisticated information system must be in place to gather the data necessary to provide quality assessments with high validity. These assessments must be based on a series of standards, developed by the professionals, against which all outcomes are measured. Recent pay-for-performance reimbursement methods have their foundation in both process and outcome quality measures. The delivery of quality care is certainly one of the principal risks, but there are a number of others; these include financial, institutional, staff, and insurance risks. Discussion of risk and uncertainty provides a foundation for consideration of managed care, which has had a significant impact on the delivery of medical services. Managed care is beginning to mature into a process that emphasizes quality and pay for performance.

Case in Point

Dr. Byrd, the chief of cardiology of a large group practice, had been charged with the responsibility of evaluating coronary artery surgery procedures. His first task was to evaluate the outcomes of patients who had undergone single-vessel bypass surgery. His studies compared those patients with similar heart conditions who were treated medically versus those who had been treated surgically with a bypass procedure. He looked at the outcomes over a period of six months, one year, and two years and found little difference in the morbidity and mortality between the two groups of patients. Further study indicated little difference in the quality of life between the groups. How should Dr. Byrd present this information to the surgeons?

Quality

A National Perspective

Quality in the U.S. healthcare system is not what it should be. A number of studies demonstrated the gaps and suggested a number of ways in which care delivery could be improved. Claude Lenfant, director of the National Heart, Lung and Blood Institute, discussed some of the shortcomings of the U.S. system (Lenfant 2003, p. 868):

> Americans spend almost 40% more for health care than any other country, yet rank 27th in infant mortality, 27th in life expectancy, and are less satisfied with their care than the English, Canadians or Germans. Serious medication errors occur in 7 of 100 hospital admissions, and more than the 80,000 unnecessary hysterectomies and 500,000 unnecessary Cesarean deliveries are performed in this country each year. Only one in five elderly myocardial infarction survivors received appropriate medications to reduce the risk of recurrence, and even fewer high risk elderly individuals are vaccinated against pneumococcus. Extensive waits and delays abounded in health care, far more than individuals tolerate in the other service sectors.

Lenfant believes health providers and members of the public are not applying what they know. This is indeed serious business.

We have known these shortcomings to be true for years based on personal stories and anecdotes. Beyond the single cases and storytelling of terrible experiences the evidence for this deficiency in quality came to light in three major reports:

1. The Institute of Medicine's (IOM) National Roundtable on Health Care Quality report, "The Urgent Need to Improve Health Care Quality" (Chassin and Galvin 1998);

2. IOM's *To Err Is Human* report (Kohn, Corrigan, and Donaldson 2000); and

3. IOM's *Crossing the Quality Chasm* report (IOM 2002).

These reports state clearly the status of quality in the U.S. healthcare system and the problems, issues, and opportunities facing providers, government, and the public.

Definition of Quality

In spite of all this the definition of quality remains somewhat elusive and seems to vacillate between the art and science of medicine (Mullan 2001). In defining quality the IOM Committee to Design a Strategy for Quality Review and Assurance in Medicare stated (Lohr 1990, p. 2).

> Quality care is the degree to which health services for individuals and populations increase the likelihood of desired health outcomes and are consistent with current professional knowledge.... How care is provided should reflect appropriate use of the most current knowledge about scientific, clinical, technical, interpersonal, manual, cognitive, and organizational managements of health care.

The definition of quality was simplified in *Crossing the Quality Chasm*, which stated, "Healthcare should be safe, effective, efficient, timely, patient centered and equitable" (IOM 2002, p. xi). These elements represent the six objectives of a quality system.

A significant relationship exists among quality, utilization review, and professional liability. A high-quality practice is much less likely to be named in a professional liability action. On the other hand an overly ambitious utilization review program with rigorous standards that may discourage physicians from ordering needed tests or procedures may increase the potential for liability action because patients may believe they have not received the necessary tests, procedures, or care. Patients may believe they should have had certain tests done that would have influenced the outcome of their care, and this may also influence their perception of quality.

Importance of Quality Perspectives

The primary responsibility for quality programs rests with the physician president or medical director of the group practice. The principal administrator is responsible for ensuring that an infrastructure for continuous quality measurement is in place. Leadership and management of the organization must understand the difference between quality in the eyes of the patient and quality in the eyes of the professionals.

The patient defines quality in the following terms:

- Was I able to get an appointment at the appropriate time?
- Was I greeted at the clinic as though I were a guest?

- Was the waiting time appropriate?
- Was the nurse or medical assistant interested in my concerns?
- Did the doctor take time with me?
- Was the doctor friendly, and did she answer all of my questions and discuss my case with me?
- Was the environment friendly, considerate, and clean?

If the responses to these questions are positive, the patient will define the care as high quality.

The professional defines quality in the following terms:

- Was the process of the patient's care provided according to the highest standards of evidence-based medicine?
- Were the appropriate protocols and guidelines for diagnosis and treatment followed?
- Were the expected outcomes for the patient's condition achieved?

Thus we see a considerable difference in the way quality is viewed by patients and healthcare providers.

Quality Assessment and Improvement

All group practices should have a quality improvement committee. It is leadership's responsibility to ensure that the committee is functioning at the highest level possible. The committee should oversee all quality improvement activities within the organization and periodically review program reports on access, process improvement, and outcomes. The group should report directly to the president and board of directors. The physicians on the committee should have the responsibility of establishing the practice standards for the organization.

The size and complexity of the quality improvement committee should be consistent with that of the organization. Specifically the charge given to the committee by the board of directors should be to:

- develop a measurement philosophy;
- identify the concepts to be measured;
- select specific indicators;
- develop operational definitions for each indicator;
- develop a data collection plan and gather the data;
- analyze the data using statistical process control; and
- use the results to increase the quality of care delivered (Lloyd 2004).

Management Perspective

The manager is primarily responsible for the development of an infrastructure that will support the group practice's quality assessment program. The foundation of that infrastructure resides in the information system and the organization's ability to develop meaningful analyses for the evaluation of process, structure, and outcome. As the old saw tells us, "You cannot manage what you cannot measure." It is incumbent on the manager and management team to ensure that measuring tools are in place regardless of what methodology might be used to evaluate the practice's quality.

Ward (2004) suggested that organizations adopt a two-tiered vision that involves information systems to establish best practices and provide performance reporting. Without a significant information infrastructure, achieving that vision is an impossible task. It comes down to choosing the right things and then doing the right things right.

Staff Education

Staff, including physicians, must understand what quality evaluation is all about and how it reflects on the care delivered to patients. While strong direction and leadership are needed, dedication and involvement at all levels of management are critical. Regular education sessions should be held with members of the management staff as well as those who deliver care. Quality is essential to the success of the organization; it is also a key factor in mitigating the risks the organization faces on a daily basis. An environment that does not promote quality assessment, evaluation, and emprovement is a risky environment. Things can easily go wrong and often do in organizations that do not evaluate quality on a consistent basis. Therefore, the organization must have methods for evaluating both quality and risk at all levels. The uncertainty surrounding that risk must also be evaluated.

Risk and Uncertainty

All organizations are at risk in a variety of areas. It is important that managers have tools in place to evaluate risk and mitigate it insofar as it is possible. "Risk is potential variation in outcomes. When risk is present, outcomes cannot be forecasted with certainty. As a result risk gives rise to uncertainty" (Williams, Smith, and Young 1998, p. 4). Each day as the manager goes about his tasks he is faced with both risk and uncertainty. This risk may involve quality issues, professional liability, finance, physical assets, general liability, or human assets. Table 9.1 shows the risks and their associated control measures.

In order to deal with these risks and decrease the amount of uncertainty the manager is responsible for the development and implementation of a risk-control program.

A risk-control program involves ongoing evaluation of the multiple risks facing the organization. An incident reporting system documents those

TABLE 9.1
Risk and
Controls

Risk Area	Risk-control Measures
Quality	Quality assessment and improvement committee, quality evaluation process
Professional Liability	Incident reporting system and insurance
Finance	Budget and financial reporting systems, contract evaluation
Physical Assets	Ongoing maintenance and insurance
General Liability	Incident reporting system, maintenance, insurance
Human Assets	Human resources policies, conflict resolution process, insurance

things that happen in an organization that could increase its risk and therefore its liabilities. The incident reporting system must cover all facets of the organization's activities and be as sensitive as possible to the environment. The incident reporting system, which should be defined by policy and the results yielded by the system, should be evaluated on a quarterly basis. Any change in incident levels must be noted and investigated promptly. This is not only true for professional liability issues but all other risks facing the organization as well. There is significant risk in managing the patient care aspects of the system, but all other risk potentials such as employee, financial, liability and disaster, also ought to be included.

On some occasions the risk is difficult to mitigate and the degree of uncertainty is high. It is important in these situations to be able to ensure the risk and potential loss at a level commensurate with the degree of uncertainty.

Another form of risk the group practice must deal with efficiently involves the insurance contracts and managed care organizations (MCOs) that insure the practice's patients. It is important to understand managed care not only from in terms of its insurance principles but in terms of its philosophy and influence on the quality of the healthcare delivery.

Managed Care

Managed care has its roots in the early 1970s, when legislation was passed giving birth to health maintenance organizations (HMOs). HMOs were predicated on an insurance plan that had capitation (payment to the provider of a certain sum per person per month) as the method of reimbursement, community rating (all groups pay the same premium), open enrollment (at least once a year occurs a period during which anyone can join), and no exclusions for existing disease. The HMO was to concentrate on prevention and health maintenance.

The competitive market did not allow the idea of the HMO to mature, and in its place evolved the MCO, which retained some but not all of the characteristics of the HMO. Qualified HMOs were required to have community rating, open enrollment, and no exclusions from pre-existing conditions. Thus the insurers could skim the good risks with low premiums, leaving the high risk to the HMO. Capitation is still found in some areas of the United States, primarily California. The principal criticism of capitation is that it may influence physicians to provide less care because the prepaid rate may not cover all of a patient's care, creating an incentive to undertreat.

Another problem was capitation rates as they were applied to primary care physicians compared to other medical and surgical specialties. Many capitated plans paid capitation to primary care physicians with the expectation that they would pay for specialty care needed by their patients out of this amount. That approach was unsuccessful, so the MCOs paid a separate capitation rate for primary and specialty care. The determination of the capitation rates, however, turned out to be an extremely difficult process, leading many plans to move back to other forms of reimbursement, especially discounted fee-for-service and relative value systems.

Although the term managed care did not find its way into the language of healthcare until the early 1980s, the notion of containing costs was certainly part of the philosophy of health maintenance. A number of definitions of managed care exist, and the one that seems most applicable is a system designed to control the utilization of healthcare and pass the risk on to the provider. Another way of looking at managed care is as the interface between the economics of care and the delivery system itself. Put in simple terms managed care was born to control cost. The concept, however, has been maturing since the end of the twentieth century, and managed care now appears to be headed in the direction of ensuring access, care management, and quality.

More recently MCOs have been involved with the development of pay-for-performance measures through which organizations that are successful with processes such as quality assessment and disease management will be rewarded; those who do not have such programs in place will not receive the benefits.

Implications for Management

There are a host of implications managers must consider, not the least of which is the ability to contract with MCOs to provide services to the MCO's enrollees. Often these contracts are extremely complicated; in order to do well financially it is important that managers understand every clause in the contract. Negotiating managed care contracts is a professional activity and must involve both physicians and managers (Kongstvedt 2001). Scrutiny by the group's general counsel is also a critical aspect of managed care contracting.

MCOs prefer negotiating contracts with smaller groups, where they have significant leverage. Negotiating with large multispecialty groups can be a problem because of the strength in numbers and the ability to deliver a broad array of services with the potential for higher utilization. It is not uncommon for MCOs to place such a practice "at risk" by establishing either a capitation rate (fixed payment per member per month) or withhold. If the charges to the MCO exceed a certain level, the withhold is not paid. Should the charges to the organization be lower than predicted the withhold is paid to the physician organization. This is the most common type of risk arrangement between MCOs and group practices (see Box 9.1 for an example).

Preferred Provider Organizations (PPOs) and Independent Practice Associations (IPAs)

There are a number of different approaches to this form of putting the provider and or the patient at risk. The PPO is a concept born in the early 1980s to afford physicians not necessarily in a group the opportunity to participate as a group in a contract with an MCO or other insurer. The PPO operates largely through a system of discounts from providers and copayments paid by the patient. If the patient seeks healthcare outside of the PPO, she may have a copayment of 40 percent, whereas the payment within the PPO would be 20 percent. Emergent care, however, is generally covered at the 20 percent level even if that care is delivered outside the system.

The IPA is a group of physicians organized solely for the purpose of contracting with MCOs. There is minimal organizational structure, and the members pay a fee to participate in the organization. The group is managed through a common entity that may manage a number of IPAs. Great care must be taken by these organizations to avoid violations of the antitrust laws and regulations. The IPA usually offers discounted services, and there may be

BOX 9.1

It is estimated that the provider will charge $150,000 for services, and this level is set as the maximum.

Each month 10 percent of the provider's charges are withheld.

At the end of the year the charges exceeded the maximum by $15,000; therefore, none of the withhold is paid to the provider.

or

At the end of the year the charges made by the provider are $135,000; therefore, the withhold is paid to the provider.

a risk pool that can be distributed if the services provided or charges made fall below certain levels.

As MCOs and reimbursement systems have evolved over the past several years there has been a move from the withhold to a pay-for-performance system. If the practice meets certain agreed-on requirements for quality and process improvements and the physicians in the group are actively involved in disease management, demand management, and case management payments for services are increased even though the two latter functions are performed in the hospital.

Care Management Initiatives

Disease management is a process in which patients' chronic diseases or conditions (e.g., hypertension, diabetes) are carefully controlled through measurements and active treatment. Patients are monitored carefully, and if the practice can demonstrate that blood pressure levels in the case of hypertension or glucose levels in the case of diabetes can be controlled over a long period, it is rewarded. The theory is that careful control will reduce morbidity, mortality, and cost. A number of demonstration projects are being undertaken by the Centers for Medicare & Medicaid Services (CMS) to more fully assess the cost impact of disease management programs. MCOs may require participating group practices to develop demand management and case management programs as well.

Disease Management

Demand management is a process that places the patient in the right care situation at the earliest possible time, making it advantageous to the clinic to provide the most efficient and effective care. It has also found great value in the hospital. In many instances demand management has reduced the number of patients seeking primary care in the emergency room. The process is carried out by triage nurses who are specially trained to ensure that patients are admitted to the appropriate place in the system depending on their care requirements. Thus patients can be seen more efficiently and effectively whether they are outpatients or inpatients.

Demand Management

Case management is generally conducted while the patient is in the hospital and is especially important in situations in which the patient has multiple systemic diseases or significant multiple trauma. Case management involves specially trained nurses who follow patients while they are in the hospital under the care of different specialty physicians. The nurse serves as a coordinator of the patient's care and ensures that all appropriate information is shared by the members of the healthcare team. In general, case management reduces the length of hospitalization as well as the duplication of services.

Case Management

In some hospitals this function is being taken over by a new specialty, the physician hospitalist. These specially trained physicians work exclusively in the hospital setting. The thought is that the patients will be under continuous on-site care and the patient's regular physician will be able to spend time more efficiently in the clinic setting.

The Future of Managed Care

It is difficult to offer a clear statement about the future of managed care. What is clear, however, is that managed care has had significant impact and is today serving as the foundation for the development of a new emphasis on quality and operational efficiency. We may see a shift away from strict cost control and discounts to more efficient delivery of care (especially outpatient); the emergence of pay-for-performance activities and demonstrations is evidence that managed care is moving in that direction.

The assumption that increased performance leads to higher quality and lower cost is now being tested. Virtually all of the organizations participating in the CMS demonstrations are group practices.

Summary

Quality assessment and improvement are key and critical to medical practice. The process, structure, and outcome of medical care can be measured in a number of ways. Leadership and management of the group practice must have an active program in place for ensuring quality. Quality improvement involves a variety of risks in the care environment, and the manager must have in place a comprehensive risk evaluation and control program to protect patients and the organization. Part of the risk-uncertainty equation is the process of contracting with MCOs and other types of insurers. More and more these organizations are demanding that providers demonstrate quality assessment and improvement programs. Thus a strong relationship exists among quality, risk, and managed care; this relationship must be understood by the manager in the group practice setting. Managed care is being transformed from a purely cost-cutting philosophy to pay for performance with the assumption that high performance will lead to high quality and lower cost.

Discussion Questions

1. What is quality in the eyes of the patient as well as from the perspective of the professional?

2. What are the key tenets found in the IOM report *Crossing the Quality Chasm*?
3. What are the responsibilities of the manager in the development of a quality assessment program in the group practice?
4. What place does pay for performance have in the managed care environment?
5. How are quality and risk related to managed care?

References

Chassin, M. R., and R. W. Galvin. 1998. "The Urgent Need to Improve Health Care Quality. Institute of Medicine National Roundtable on Health Care Quality." *Journal of the American Medical Association* 280 (11): 1000–1005.

Institute of Medicine. 2002. *Crossing the Quality Chasm: The IOM Health Care Quality Initiative.* [Online information; retrieved 02/22/05.] www.iom.edu/view.asp?id=8089.

Kohn, L. T., M. Corrigan, and M. S. Donaldson (Eds.). Committee on Quality of Health Care in America, Institute of Medicine. 2000. *To Err Is Human: Building a Safer Health System.* [Online information; retrieved 02/22/05.] www.nap.edu/books/0309068371/html/.

Kongstvedt, P. R. (Ed.). 2001. *Essentials of Managed Health Care.* Gaithersburg, MD: Aspen Publishers.

Lenfant, C. 2003. "Shattuck Lecture—Clinical Research to Clinical Practice—Lost in Translation?" *New England Journal of Medicine* 349 (9): 868–74.

Lloyd, R. C. 2004. "The Search for a Few Good Indicators." In *The Healthcare Quality Book: Vision, Strategy, and Tools*, edited by S. B. Ransom, M. Joshi, and D. B. Nash, pp. 89–115. Chicago: Health Administration Press.

Lohr, K. N. (Ed.). 1990. *Medicare: A Strategy for Quality Assurance, Vol. I.* Washington, D.C.: Institute of Medicine, National Academy Press.

Mullan, F. 2001. "A Founder of Quality Assessment Encounters a Troubled System Firsthand." *Health Affairs* 20 (1): 137–41.

Ward, R. E. 2004. "Information Technology Applications for Improved Quality." In *The Healthcare Quality Book: Vision, Strategy, and Tools*, edited by S. B. Ransom, M. Joshi, and D. B. Nash, pp. 267–307. Chicago: Health Administration Press.

Williams, C. A., M. L. Smith, and P. C. Young. 1998. *Risk Management and Insurance, 8th Edition.* Boston: Irwin McGraw-Hill.

Wyszewianski, L. 2004. "Basic Concepts of Healthcare Quality." In *The Healthcare Quality Book: Vision, Strategy, and Tools*, edited by S. B. Ransom, M. Joshi, and D. B. Nash, pp. 25–40. Chicago: Health Administration Press.

Suggested Readings

Berwick, D. M. 2002. "A User's Guide for the IOM's 'Quality Chasm' Report." *Health Affairs* 21 (3): 80–90.

Chassin, M. R. 1998. "Is Health Care Ready for Six Sigma Quality?" *The Milbank Quarterly* 76 (4): 565–91.

Eddy, D. M. 1998. "Performance Measurement: Problems and Solutions." *Health Affairs* 17 (4): 7–25.

Ettinger, W. H. 2001. "Six Sigma: Applying GE's Lessons to Health Care." *Trustee* 54 (8): 10–15.

Inamdar, N., R. S. Kaplan, and M. Bower. 2002. "Applying the Balanced Scorecard in Healthcare Provider Organizations." *Journal of Healthcare Management* 47 (3): 179–95.

Kaplan, R. S., and D. P. Norton. 1996. "Using the Balanced Scorecard as a Strategic Management System." *Harvard Business Review* 74 (1): 75–85.

Wennberg, J. E. 2002. "Unwarranted Variations in Healthcare Delivery: Implications for Academic Medical Centres." *British Medical Journal* 325 (7370): 961–64.

PHYSICIAN-HOSPITAL RELATIONSHIPS

Joseph W. Mitlyng

Learning Objectives

This chapter will enable the reader to:

- identify the relative stability in physician-hospital relations that existed for decades prior to the early 1990s and the major continuing changes in those relationships that have occurred since;
- identify common examples of current physician-hospital relationships;
- gain an overview of the regulatory and legal considerations that frame the environment for physician-hospital relationships;
- grasp the different perspectives that physicians and hospital leadership bring to these relationships;
- understand the potential for conflict as the captain of the ship meets the leader of the corporation;
- identify common physician values, hospital leadership values, and shared values; and
- realize the potential for collaborative strategic relationships between partners as a model for future physician-hospital relationships.

Chapter Purpose

This chapter provides an understanding of present physician-hospital relationships in the context of the history of these relationships, the regulatory and legal environment, and differing perspectives of physicians and hospitals. The chapter outlines the values held by many physicians, the values held by many hospital leaders, and the ways in which some physicians and hospitals are building on shared values to develop collaborative strategic partnerships. These partnerships are built on mutual trust and engage physicians and hospitals in each other's success.

CASE IN POINT

John Daniels was in his second week as the new CEO of Memorial Hospital, a 400-bed community hospital. The hospital had an operating margin of 0.5 percent of revenue in the previous fiscal year. The previous CEO had been with the hospital for many years, and John knew that part of his work this first year was going to have to be to take a hard look at costs.

In the previous hour John had met with Dr. Bill Swift, the leader of a 30-physician internal medicine group that was a major admitter of patients to the hospital. Dr. Swift had asked if the hospital might be interested in selling the group block time on its MRI machine for its patients. The hospital was currently performing those scans, billing for them, and making the profit on them. Dr. Swift noted that he had heard of hospitals in other areas of the country selling these services to physician practices as an industrial account that enabled the practice to bill for the services and make a profit on them. He had not talked with St. Michael's Hospital, the other area hospital; he first wanted to talk with John about the possibility of buying block MRI time from Memorial.

John had said that he would talk with his staff and see what might be done. They agreed to meet in a week to talk again. John began to think about the issues involved. What are the negative and positive issues, and what should John do?

History of Physician-Hospital Relationships

The following phases describe four different periods in the evolution of physician-hospital relationships. The years associated with the different periods reflect the time of these changes for much of the United States, but they are only to provide a general reference for the reader. The timing of the phases has differed, with some areas of the country leading these changes and others coming to them later.

Prior to the Early 1990s

Prior to the 1990s physicians and hospitals were generally separate independent entities. Physicians hospitalized their patients when hospital care was needed. Some specialists, such as anesthesiologists, worked only in the hospital, but physicians and hospitals saw each other as quite different, independent businesses. Services were seen as either hospital- or physician-provided services. With the exception of a few large medical groups with the size and resources to add CT scanners and advanced laboratory testing, there was little competition between physicians and hospitals to provide the same services.

A limited number of exceptions in this period had early in their history developed as combined physician groups and hospitals (e.g., Geisinger Health System, Scott & White, Virginia Mason). Kaiser Permanente in California was a case by itself, with its combined organization including a physician group, hospitals, and prepaid health insurance.

Early 1990s to Mid-1990s

Managed care had its beginnings in the Midwest and California. Prior to Paul Ellwood, MD, coining the phrase health maintenance organizations (HMOs) and the passage of the HMO Act of 1973, large medical groups in the Midwest (e.g., Marshfield Clinic, Park Nicollet Clinic) started prepaid insurance plans as a way of helping patients pay their bills. Group Health in Minneapolis provided care to its enrollees through its employed physician group. Managed care plans became an economic force in healthcare in Minneapolis and Los Angeles in the mid-1980s. The mid-1980s to mid-1990s saw the expansion of managed care plans as an economic force across the country.

The proposal of the Clinton healthcare plan in 1992 brought with it a strong conviction in the minds of many healthcare leaders that nationalized healthcare, based on accountable health plans organizing and providing managed care, was about to be a reality. Examples were already in operation. Kaiser Permanente was seen as the early archetype of what came to be known as an integrated delivery system (IDS), but there were similar organizations in the Midwest in which large multispecialty groups, working with their affiliated hospitals, were close to being full IDSs as well.

The conclusion was clear: IDSs would be required to compete in this new healthcare environment of accountable health plans. Some multispecialty physician group–hospital health systems were already affiliated as noted above and had also developed HMOs as part of their systems. Other multispecialty groups, such as Park Nicollet Medical Center, made plans to merge with their primary hospitals. Hospitals merged with or acquired major physician groups and competed aggressively to recruit primary care physicians. The theory behind this recruiting was that without the physician base the hospitals would be shut out of managed care contracts and out of business; furthermore, managing care well would save so much money that the cost paid to acquire the practices was close to irrelevant.

Physician practice management companies (PPMCs) were also developed to acquire and manage physician practices. The theory behind these organizations was that size would be required to negotiate reasonable reimbursement rates and by developing a large network the PPMCs would be able to dictate substantially better rates. The PPMCs were also convinced that their superior professional management skills would enable them to reduce practice costs, continue to pay their physicians a competitive salary, and produce an ongoing income stream to reward their investors. This experiment, however, proved to be for the most part successful.

Mid-1990s to Early 2000s

After the defeat of the Clinton plan came a backlash by the public and purchasers of health insurance against the restrictions of managed care. The health insurers turned to more open physician and hospital networks to attract patients to their products. The convincing line was, "Your doctor is in our network."

When the managed care requirement and value of managing care did not occur, insurers turned to decreases in physician and hospital unit reimbursement rates to produce profits. The decline in reimbursement coupled with high base salary commitments to physicians and inflated investments made to acquire practices led to large losses by hospitals. Many hospitals chose to divest the employed physician practices to eliminate the ongoing operating losses from these practices.

The PPMCs filed for bankruptcy. Their theory that a large network would guarantee good rates from insurers proved false; what counted was the degree of competition in each local area. The physician groups realized that their clout with payers was the same as the market position the group had enjoyed before joining the PPMC, and groups could see no market value for the fees they were committed to pay the PPMCs. The theory that the PPMCs could substantially reduce the costs of practice through superior management also proved false. The PPMCs learned that although opportunities existed, they were not as great as anticipated. Private physician practices are typically small businesses run by the physicians who are part of the practice. Like other small business owners, physicians want control.

In contrast to the general divestment of physician practices some hospitals and health systems chose to keep their employed physician groups and improve their performance, as discussed below.

Early 2000s to Present

Insurers have a stronger position than hospitals and physicians in many markets. Insurers have been able to hold down payment increases and in some specialties actually decrease the amounts paid to physicians. Advancing technology has blurred the lines between hospital and physician services. Cataract surgery, for instance, once required a 14-day hospital stay with the patient in bed, head immobilized with sandbags; today this is an outpatient procedure. To maintain or increase their income physicians are developing services in direct competition with hospitals.

There is growing recognition of the need for collaborative relationships between physicians and hospitals. Some believe physicians are interested only in increasing their compensation, but other drivers for physicians are control of the practice environment and efficiency of practice. Working well with physicians requires addressing all of their values and interests. An early example that recognized physician values of control, efficiency, and a share of the financial return occurred in 1992 when one hospital system built an outpatient surgery unit and handed it over to physicians to run, with the hospital receiving a percentage of the unit's profit (Francis 2004).

Hospitals with employed physician groups have continued their efforts to improve the performance of their groups. These hospitals and health systems have developed effective leadership teams that manage the employed physician group as if it were an independent medical group accountable for its financial performance. Hospitals with strong employed physician groups (significant size in the market with a strong leadership team) have found these groups to be strategic partners in dealing with insurance companies. If a hospital refuses an insurer's contract and does not have an employed physician group, the patients will be admitted to a competing hospital. If a hospital with a strong employed physician group refuses a contract, the physicians and hospital will lose some patients, but the insurer will also lose some enrollees as patients choose to stay with their physicians; this uncertainty improves the negotiation. These strong physician groups are now attracting some prestigious private practices that see advantages in joining large, successful hospital-based groups.

Examples of Physician-Hospital Relationships

The following sections present examples of physician-hospital relationships today. Some relationships, such as membership in the hospital's medical staff, predate by decades the changes that have occurred since the early 1990s. Others, such as joint ventures, became more common in response to those changes.

Member of the Hospital Medical Staff

The rights and responsibilities of the hospital medical staff illustrate a "linked yet separate" relationship between hospitals and the physicians on staff. The medical staff organization is responsible for the quality of care provided by physicians, and hospitals are legally required to have a medical staff organization independent of hospital leadership. The medical staff, which reports to the board of the hospital, is a formal organization with its own bylaws and officers. The medical staff organization is responsible for the credentialing of new physicians and for making recommendations to the board for granting or revoking privileges.

The medical staff functions are independent of hospital leadership, but in an effective organization a close working relationship exists. The hospital provides support staff for the medical staff, and the hospital CEO brings the reports of the medical staff to the board. A voluntary, not-for-profit hospital is most effective when the influence of the board, hospital leadership, and medical staff are in balance, like a tripartite form of government. The board is the legislative function; hospital leadership is the executive branch; and the medical staff is the judicial branch. They are independent but rely on one another for success. The key is in the balance of power and the relationships, each part doing its own job in an integrated manner.

All physicians in clinical practice are members of the medical staff, whether they are employed by the hospital or in independent practice. Members of the medical staff may work only with one hospital or have privileges at multiple hospitals.

Employment by the Hospital

A second physician-hospital relationship is direct employment by the hospital. Some physicians are employed to fill leadership positions (e.g., chief medical officer) that are part of and accountable to hospital leadership. The positions of chiefs of service are filled on a voluntary basis in smaller hospitals, but in larger hospitals and those with teaching programs these positions are employed physician leadership positions.

Physicians are also employed by hospitals to provide clinical care. They may be employed directly by the hospital or by a physician group owned by the hospital.

Contractual Relationship with the Hospital

Some physician groups are typically in independent private practice but have an exclusive relationship with one or more hospitals. Common examples are anesthesiology, emergency, radiology, and pathology physician groups. In a contractual relationship the hospital defines the relationship—the work required—and the group agrees to perform as required by the contract.

Joint Ventures

In a joint venture the hospital and physicians (typically a group of physicians) maintain their organizational independence. Many different labels may be applied, but the essential feature is working together to achieve the separate objectives of the hospital and physician group. Joint ventures require agreements on shared governance; agreements on equity investment and sharing of profits or losses; and a leadership and management team accountable to the joint venture partners. (See Chapter 3 for a discussion of different forms of partnership in medical group practice.)

Overview of Regulatory and Legal Considerations

Potential legal issues arise with all of the above relationships, as described in this section.

Four sets of laws and related regulations set boundaries on permissible actions for physicians and hospitals. A healthcare executive needs to understand the general applicability of each of these areas to possible decisions and actions. This section provides the reader with an awareness of the issues to know what may apply—and when to call in a healthcare lawyer to assist in developing or reviewing proposed agreements to ensure appropriate compliance.

Antitrust Laws (Sherman, FTC, and Clayton Acts)

The antitrust laws and regulations prohibit monopolies or joint actions with otherwise independent physicians or hospitals that have the effect of unreasonably reducing competition and increasing prices in a market. Price fixing, the action by otherwise independent practices to set fees, is considered a violation in all cases. In other cases the question of what constitutes unreasonable activity is subject to review and judgment.

Physicians in independent practices, for example, are generally prohibited from acting together to:

- refuse to accept a proposed fee schedule from a payer;
- merge so all physicians in a specialty in the service area are in one group; or
- vote to refuse hospital staff privileges for a new physician if that means the physician will not be able to practice in the service area.

Violation of the Sherman antitrust law is a felony punishable by fines of up to $10 million for corporations or $350,000 for individuals, or by imprisonment of up to three years for both.

The Federal Trade Commission's (FTC) Web site (www.FTC.gov) is a good source for added information on the antitrust laws and current examples of the FTC's application of those laws. FTC provides advisory opinions with respect to a specific course of proposed action.

Stark I and II (Section 1877, Social Security Act)

The Stark laws were developed in response to the concern that physician referrals for services in which the physician has a financial relationship would lead to unnecessary utilization of those services and unnecessary increases in the cost to care for Medicare patients. The services covered by this prohibition are referred to as designated health services (DHS). The Stark laws prohibit referral by physicians of Medicare patients to DHS owned by themselves or members of their families—either directly or as part of an ownership group—or where there is a financial relationship by contract.

The group practice exemption says that physicians practicing as a group can own these DHS, such as laboratory and radiology services, as a group. The group's internal compensation system, however, cannot reward individual physician members of the group for the volume or value of these referred services. The profit on the referred services must be treated as group profit and used to offset the costs of the group as a whole.

An overriding theme in the Stark law is that contract relationships between physicians and hospitals must be structured at fair market value and be legitimate business transactions in the absence of referral considerations. The value of external considerations that can be seen as compensation must be considered as part of the fair market value calculation. Examples of these forms of compensation include leases, medical directorships, recruitment subsidies, and service contracts. The theme of fair market value transactions is a major element of the laws and regulations affecting physician-hospital relationships and will be discussed further below.

The regulations provide other safe harbors in addition to the group practice exemption that may be helpful in a specific situation.

According to the Centers for Medicare & Medicaid Services (CMS), the penalties for violation of the Stark laws are as follows:

- Failure to report covered services (DHS) provided by the group incurs a civil monetary penalty of not more than $10,000 per day for which reporting is required to be made (CMS 2004, p. 17933).
- Claims for DHS provided as a result of a prohibited referral will not be paid, and payments for any such claims must be refunded; individuals and entities that knowingly violate the prohibition are also subject to civil monetary penalties (CMS 2004, p. 17934).

The CMS Web site (www.CMS.gov) is the source for information on the Stark law and related CMS regulations. Related associations, such as the Medical Group Management Association (www.MGMA.com) also provide extensive information on the Stark law and regulations.

Medicare and Medicaid Antikickback Statute (Section 1128, Social Security Act)

The antikickback statute prohibits the knowing and willful offer to pay (or receive) financial incentives to a physician to induce him to: (1) refer patients for services; or (2) obtain or recommend obtaining a good or service that will be paid for by Medicare or Medicaid. The incentives prohibited may be in any form that has a financial benefit to the physician, including direct or indirect payments. Indirect payments can be any other financial transaction that provides financial benefit to the physician, such as payments above market value for space owned by the physician or the lease of equipment to the physician at less than the cost of that equipment.

The penalties for violating the antikickback statute include both civil monetary and criminal penalties. Enforcement of this statute falls under the joint responsibility of the Department of Health and Human Services and Department of Justice. The Department of Justice's Web site (www.DOJ.gov) is a good source for added information on the statute and advisory opinions that have been issued. The Department of Health and Human Services (in consultation with the Department of Justice) provides formal, written advisory opinions on the application of the antikickback statute and the safe harbor provisions (U.S. Department of Justice 1998).

Inurement and Private Benefit (IRS Code, Section 4958)

Hospitals and/or clinics classified as not-for-profit organizations for federal tax purposes are known as 501(c)(3) tax-exempt organizations, referencing the tax code section that governs their not-for-profit status. Organizations with 501(c)(3) status are required to direct their activities exclusively for charitable, educational, or other public-good benefits for the community. None of the earnings of the organization may inure to any private individual. (Inurement is said to have occurred when an officer or other person considered an insider receives excess benefit, such as unreasonably high compensation, from the organization. Private benefit is excessive benefit to individuals outside the organization.)

Inurement and private benefit carry the potential loss of tax-exempt status, but this penalty is so severe that the IRS developed intermediate sanction regulations that provide the following penalties:

- The individual receiving the excess benefit is required to return the amount of the excess benefit plus pay a 25 percent tax on the amount.
- If the individual receiving the excess benefit does not return the amount of the excess benefit to the organization by the earlier of the time the individual is notified of the determination or assessment of the 25 percent tax, the individual is taxed an additional 200 percent of the excess benefit.
- Managers (including officers and board members) who knowingly approved of the transaction are subject to a 10 percent tax on the excess benefit up to $10,000 for each excess benefit transaction.

A safe harbor exists for organizational managers if the organization obtains a "reasoned opinion of counsel" that the transaction is reasonable. This step will avoid the potential 10 percent tax for knowingly approving the transaction.

The laws and regulations proscribing the activities and relationships of physicians and hospitals are significant, and the penalties for violating those laws and regulations are substantial. It is important to focus on developing services and relationships between physicians and hospitals that provide better care for patients, a competitive source for care in the community, and referrals for services based on best medical judgment rather than individual economic self-interest. This section is not to be used as a substitute for competent legal advice; to the contrary, the points in this section should make clear that an experienced healthcare lawyer should be retained and consulted for decisions that involve areas covered by these laws and regulations.

Physician and Hospital Perspectives

The difference in perspectives has both patient care and financial components. Physicians see the hospital as one of the places they provide care to patients. The hospital is a place of work with specialized staff, equipment (diagnostic testing and surgical equipment), and facilities (operating rooms and hospital rooms) that are expected to help them care for patients. The physician is the captain of the ship in directing the use of the hospital's resources to care for her patients. By practice and law the physician is responsible for the overall direction of care for her patients.

Hospital CEOs, on the other hand, see the hospital as a place where people in their service area come for the services provided by the hospital. Physicians in the hospital are an important part of the services provided by the hospital, but only a part. The hospital staff includes all staff who are not physicians, and the medical staff includes all physicians. The hospital CEO is responsible for the financial performance of the hospital, and although individual physicians may be interested in and concerned about the hospital's financial performance, it is not their responsibility.

Hospital CEOs see themselves as responsible for the quality of care provided by anyone who has professional contact with patients in the hospital. One CEO required anyone who had contact with patients in the hospital to be credentialed: The city ministerial association credentialed all of the clergy; vendor representatives who might come in contact with patients had to sign contracts that defined the limits of what they could do in the hospital; and EMT technicians credentialed the emergency department assistants.

Inherent Potential for Conflict

As the captain of the ship, the physician, meets and deals with the leader of the corporation, the hospital CEO,[1] the question of who is in charge sometimes arises. One might think the physicians decide the clinical issues and hospital leadership decide the administrative issues; in reality few issues are purely clinical or administrative. Buying a piece of clinical equipment or determining the number of nurses and other staff on a unit can directly affect the physician's ability to care for his patients. Such a decision also directly affects the financial performance of the hospital.

It is important to resolve these differing viewpoints in a way that meets the reasonable needs of the physician and hospital. Failure to do so results in the physician not getting what he needs to care for his patients. Hospital leaders who fall into a pattern of not resolving differences and meeting the reasonable needs of physicians risk a vote of no confidence by the medical staff, and continued failure results in eventual termination by the hospital board.

Value Systems

The key to resolving differing viewpoints in a reasonable way is finding common ground in shared values, vision, strategies, and benefits. Each physician and hospital leader has a unique set of values, with differing relative importance for each value. That said, there are values held by most physicians and values held by most hospital leaders, and the two groups share many values. Shared values provide the basis for developing a shared vision and shared strategies that produce mutual benefit.

Physician Values

Physicians will make choices they see are in the best interests of their patients and themselves. Looking at the decision to be made as purely one of maximizing dollar return is a mistake in working with most physicians. Physicians are often viewed as highly motivated by money, but the reality is a far more complex set of interests and values (Mitlyng and Wenzel 1999) that include the following, as stated in chaper two.

1. **Providing the best care for their patients**. This is the fundamental value of physicians. It is the original drive that provides sustained satisfaction.
2. **Personal control over what they do and how they practice**. Physicians are trained to be in charge. They are held responsible, both legally and by their profession, for what does or does not happen to patients under their care.
3. **Limited control by others**. This is a corollary to the above point. Control is acceptable only in areas where others clearly have the responsibility and more expertise. For most physicians billing and collections, accounting and finance, computer systems, human resources management, and contract negotiation are examples of these areas. Decisions in other areas may be made with the best intentions, but until physicians understand and accept them, those decisions are seen as limits on the first and second points.
4. **Doing well in comparison with peers**. Doing well on report cards is part of the experience of becoming a physician, and comparisons with others are always seen as report cards.

5. **Sense of fairness in relationships**. Even tough decisions are acceptable if they result from an open and fair process. Arbitrary decisions based solely on the power of position are unacceptable.

6. **Environment of clinical inquiry**. Physicians continue to learn from their experiences and those of others to keep current with best medical practices.

7. **Opportunity for dialogue and ability to influence decisions affecting them**. Listening to and hearing the physician's perspective is critical. Data and real dialogue are valued as the basis for reaching decisions.

8. **Maintaining collegial relations with peers**. Relationships are based on working together as peers, each as professionals with special competencies.

9. **Choice of those with whom they work**. Physicians must rely on their colleagues and coworkers in caring for patients, and the quality of their colleagues and coworkers reflects on them.

Hospital Values

1. **Providing the highest quality medical care possible for patients and the community**. As with physicians, this is the fundamental drive that led to the establishment of community hospitals. This value is key in attracting physicians to hospitalize their patients at a given hospital.

2. **Developing a seamless network of care with other healthcare systems**. Hospitals want to provide patients with access to a full range of high-quality care. Physicians refer their patients where they have relationships and good experience with the specialty physicians. Hospitals value being part of a network of care with physicians collectively providing the highest quality of care. A financial relationship is not required; the value is in an effective working relationship that provides staff training and easy referral of patients.

3. **Ensuring the qualifications of those who provide care in the hospital or as part of the system**. Credentialing the qualifications of those who provide care in the hospital is an inherent part of ensuring that the hospital and those who care for patients provide the highest quality care.

4. **Doing well in comparison with peers**. Hospitals and those who practice in them are driven by the requirements for personal competence in the work they do. This value is a corollary of the requirements for personal competence.

5. **Sense of fairness in relationships**. Hospitals are an integral part of their communities. There is a substantial investment in the physical facility and in the hospital's relationships with:

   - patients;
   - employees;

- payers; and
- the community itself.

These relationships are voluntary. The only long-term relationship is one in which individuals feel they are being treated fairly. Decisions seen to be unfair to one or more of these groups result in the loss of support by those groups and eventual payback actions. Hospital leaders who have had no involvement in past decisions may marvel at physicians' long memories of past slights and injustices.

The perceptions of patients, employers, and the community are also subject to long memories. The best marketing is word of mouth as patients talk about the care they received. Improving community perception once a reputation for quality or concern for the community is lost requires more than advertising that, "We provide the highest quality care."

Marketing can improve perceptions, but it also requires actions that demonstrate benefit to the community. Demonstrating concern for the community, for example, requires developing programs that address community needs (e.g., obesity awareness, smoking-cessation programs, occupational medicine, environmental risk awareness) and then talking about how the new services are benefiting the community.

6. **Fostering teaching and research**. Teaching and research are core ways of demonstrating the hospital's commitment to provide the highest quality medical care and meet the future healthcare needs of the community. These activities attract and retain to the medical staff physicians who are interested in teaching and in providing this level of care.

7. **Serving customers and seeing all relationships as relationships with customers**. The core idea is treating everyone with respect—honoring the dignity, individuality, and rights of everyone.

   - Patients are the first customer, and meeting their needs comes first—providing a secure, caring environment for patients and families and paying particular attention to patients' rights to privacy, confidentiality, and information.
   - Physicians are customers as well as an integral part of delivering care at the hospital, and meeting physicians' needs for efficient and high-quality support is essential to providing the highest quality medical care.
   - The community is a customer, and providing value through care, services, and technology of the highest quality at the lowest possible cost shows responsibility to the community for the appropriate use of its gifts, resources, and support.
   - Employees value the opportunity to provide input on issues affecting them.

Hospitals seek and use opportunities to measure, evaluate, and continually improve customer service

8. **Seeing healthcare as a calling**. This value is seeing the healthcare leadership role as something quite satisfying beyond the financial considerations. Part of the calling is seeing the importance of addressing the needs of all customers:

   - Physicians—making sure they have all they need to provide the best care for patients.
   - Payers—providing the most efficient care at the lowest cost, not just maximizing premiums.
   - Employees—representing the interests of employees to the board; presenting board policies to employees as reasonable approaches that meet the needs of all. The key is establishing a formal process of listening to the concerns and interests of employees, including meeting with the night staff at 2:00 a.m.[2]
   - Community—serving by participation in the chamber of commerce, Rotary Club, and other community service organizations and by bringing business leaders into discussions to help them better understand healthcare and how to best meet the needs of the community.
   - Patients—doing all the rest so patients benefit.

   As a calling the work merits the best efforts of all involved.

9. **Control versus partnership relationships**. Historically many hospital CEOs saw a control relationship as necessary in dealing with physicians and others; this was a common resolution of the conflict between the leader of the corporation and captain of the ship. The shift since the mid-1990s has been to recognize the benefits of partnership relationships. As one former hospital CEO put it, "Some people are control freaks, but control is overblown as an issue. If the effort is to put the patient first, control is not an issue."

Partnership Model

The partnership model uses the concept of equal partners, with both parties contributing their skills and efforts to the success of the whole. If each partner is seen as working in the best interest of the whole, agreements will be easy to achieve. If, however, self-interest is perceived, any type of collaboration will be difficult.

Shared values provide the basis for developing shared vision and strategies that can provide mutual benefit. The steps for developing a partnership and shared values are:

1. Get past the past (long memories of past failings, often in relationships with others) through open communication about shared values.
2. Conduct dialogue on possible shared interests.

3. Identify and develop ways in which the interests of both the hospital
    and physicians can be met with shared strategies.

Key areas for common values include patient-centered service, quality,
effectiveness, efficiency, research, education, and financial viability. These values can best be addressed through thoughtful and honest dialogue, with an
eye toward focusing on patients and their needs (see Figure 10.1 on the following page).

Relationship Considerations

The following sections describe the pros and cons of hospitals and physicians
working together in different relationships to form strategic partnerships.

Formal Medical Staff Organization

The development of shared strategies involves physician and hospital leaders
working together. More and more physicians are interested in getting beyond the issues of the past and searching for joint activities. Hospital leadership is also seeking greater opportunities to work with physicians for the benefit of patients.

The medical staff is not a good vehicle for working on strategies that
apply to only some of its members. The medical staff organization includes
all members of the medical staff, and it is designed to represent the interests
of all. No decision to change will be made unless an immediate benefit to all
is perceived.

It is important to consider the interests of all members of the medical
staff in developing a shared strategy with a smaller group of physicians. Other
physicians who are members of the medical staff may have interest in the
same strategy, and they may be the ones to include in initial strategy development or in any future expansion of the strategy. Others may feel they are
being treated unfairly by not being included in the strategy; dealing with
those concerns should be part of the planning process.

One writer has described the challenge of developing a strategy that
appeals to all members of the medical staff as building an ark that serves all;
it is better to build a "flotilla" including a fishing boat, sail boat, speed boat,
and other boats (Bujak 2003). The best approach is to be open to a variety
of arrangements that work for the hospital or health system and members of
the medical staff.

Physicians Employed by Hospitals

Physicians employed by hospitals can be divided into two models. First is
the model in which physicians are treated like any other employees of the

TABLE 10.1
Shared Values
and Partnership
Model

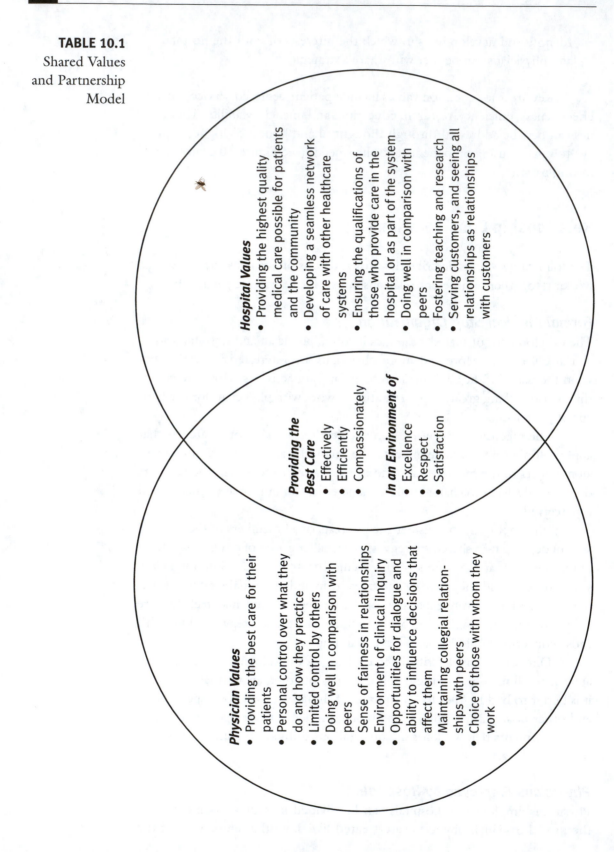

Hospital Values
- Providing the highest quality medical care possible for patients and the community
- Developing a seamless network of care with other healthcare systems
- Ensuring the qualifications of those who provide care in the hospital or as part of the system
- Doing well in comparison with peers
- Fostering teaching and research
- Serving customers, and seeing all relationships as relationships with customers

Providing the Best Care
- Effectively
- Efficiently
- Compassionately

In an Environment of
- Excellence
- Respect
- Satisfaction

Physician Values
- Providing the best care for their patients
- Personal control over what they do and how they practice
- Limited control by others
- Doing well in comparison with peers
- Sense of fairness in relationships
- Environment of clinical iInquiry
- Opportunities for dialogue and ability to influence decisions that affect them
- Maintaining collegial relation-ships with peers
- Choice of those with whom they work

hospital. This model makes the hospital responsible for the performance of its employees and has produced significant losses for employer hospitals; those losses have led to difficult relations with private practice physicians who see the hospital's assets drawn off to support the employed physicians rather than meet the needs of the private practice physicians. Compared to private practice, in which physicians and staff have an ownership interest in the care they provide to their patients, patient care and service are challenged in this environment as employees may not be motivated as they care for patients.

The second model in which physicians are employed by hospitals is more successful. Physician practices in this model are organized as a separate corporation that is owned by the hospital but has strong leadership focused on its management. The leadership team is accountable for the performance of the practice corporation and implements compensation systems in which the physicians are also accountable for the financial performance of the practice organization. Patient care and service are important values in these groups. In this model the physician group becomes much like an independent medical group affiliated with the hospital; it includes physician-administrator team leadership and management and physician governance of the practice.

Physician group authority and accountability is the significant difference between the two models. The conclusion that physician group authority and accountability for performance produce stronger physician-system alignment (and commitment to act in the best interests of the system) is consistent with a major study by Alexander et al. (2001, p. 140):

> [Our] findings support the contention made by others that formal administrative control over physician organizations is antithetical to physician values of self governance and may threaten the traditional autonomy and internalized controls exercised by physicians.... Organizational linkages should emphasize empowering physician groups to foster both authority and accountability for decisions affecting the group, rather than transferring these responsibilities to the system.

Physicians Employed by Physician Practice Management Companies (PPMCs)

PPMCs threatened to be a third party in physician-hospital relationships. They are still a factor in some specialty areas, but they have essentially disappeared as a major factor in relationships with multispecialty groups and primary care physicians. It is useful to consider what did not work in those relationships. Some factors, such as managed care contracting, can be better addressed by a major physician-community hospital partnership. The fact that physician practices have a limited profit margin after paying practice costs including competitive physician compensation holds true regardless of who owns the group.

Single-specialty PPMCs, however, have continued to have some success. Factors contributing to that success are ease of management and economies of scale. These PPMCs use compensation methods designed to keep physicians motivated by aligning incentives. Much of the purchase price is paid with contingent notes, and bonuses are paid based on productivity (Flanakin 2002).

Contractual Relationships

Contractual relationships work in defined areas such as exclusive contracts to provide specialized services in a hospital. They function well when there are common goals, the work required is clearly defined, and agreement can be reached on financial terms for the period of the contract. Contract relationships do not work well when the work is to set up a new venture (i.e., areas of responsibility are known but the work to be done is only generally defined and the benefits of the new venture can only be estimated). New ventures require collaborative, shared risk relationships.

Collaborative Relationships

Collaborative relationships are essentially partnership relationships in which both parties contribute to the joint effort and both parties benefit.

Physicians on Hospital and Health System Boards

Placing practicing physicians on hospital and health system boards (and hospital and health system leadership on physician group boards) provides a better understanding of the challenges facing each organization. This relationship increases the likelihood of the other organization's interests being taken into account in decision making, but it may actually reduce loyalty; physicians may see system membership on their board as an unwelcome intrusion and membership on the system board as only tokenism (Alexander et al. 2001). The key seems to be in how this relationship is handled by the individuals involved.

Physicians Involved in Strategic Planning and Developing New Initiatives

The value of this involvement is the potential it provides for moving ahead with collaborative relationships to jointly develop new initiatives. As with the board membership noted above, the involvement may be seen as a significant involvement leading to joint efforts or as unproductive tokenism.

Strategic Relationships Between Partners

Strategic relationships are long-term relationships. The parties to a strategic relationship want to make good choices in deciding on partners, choosing others with shared values, shared interest in the strategy, and shared interest in a long-term relationship.

Partners do not own each other. They come together and work together as long as doing so is in the interests of both. Each partner needs to take responsibility for contributing to the success of the other.

Hospitals and physicians have many strategic interests. Hospitals want to develop strategic physician relationships that stabilize the hospital's relationship with the physicians who use it. Hospitals have an interest in maintaining the financial viability of both the hospital and, within the bounds of the related laws and regulations, the practices of physicians who use the hospital.

Physicians want to increase revenue sources to offset decreases in third-party reimbursement and increases in staff and other operating costs. Physicians also want the hospital to have the staffing, equipment, and facilities needed to provide the best care for their patients.

Strategic relationships between partners require agreement on:

- shared vision and the strategy to accomplish it;
- how the investment required will be shared;
- alignment of financial risk and decision making;
- leadership and management responsibility—individuals must have the responsibility and authority required to lead and manage the joint venture and be accountable for that performance; and
- shared governance and oversight of each party's performance.

Following are two examples of strategic arrangements that are working.

Industrial Accounts

The core idea is in selling to physicians at a fair market value hospital-based services (e.g., laboratory, radiology) that the physicians can then provide for their patients and bill to third parties. Leasing block time is a related idea.

The value of this idea is that it is a way for physicians and hospitals to share resources to provide services to patients. The hospital retains a fair market value pricing for providing the service, and the practice avoids the capital investment required to set up its own services (Jones 2002).

Joint Venture Services

The example presented earlier in this chapter—of a hospital that built a medical office building with an ambulatory surgery unit and turned it over to physicians to run—illustrates the ability of hospitals and physicians to come together to meet the needs of all. This approach provides better care for patients with the new services, meets the financial needs of physicians and the hospital, meets the interests of physicians in managing the efficiency of their practices, and—compared to setting up competing ambulatory services—meets the needs of employers, payers, and the community for high-quality, cost-effective care. Other examples of joint ventures that have worked well include laboratories, imaging facilities, catheterization laboratories, isotope laboratories, and health plans.

Alternatives to Strategic Partnerships

Competition for Revenue Streams

The development of competing ambulatory surgery units, radiology and pathology testing services, and specialty hospitals demonstrates the ample opportunity to develop competing services. Hospitals have historically been a good source for capital investment, but the development of capital partners interested in investing in healthcare has provided a competing source for financing. Ample evidence shows that a good business plan for developing a healthcare service that will be profitable in competition with the local hospital can be developed and financed without involving the hospital.

The challenge for hospital and physician leadership is to look for solutions that are best for both. Organizational leaders are much like combat fighter pilots. They can take their organizations up, down, and sideways. They are always looking for opportunities to avoid threats and make themselves and their organizations more successful. Leaders of organizations also face a significant risk known as target fixation. For fighter pilots target fixation occurs when they become so focused on their mark that they fly right into it; they lose perspective and either ignore or literally do not see that the strategy they are following is not working and needs to be changed (Mitlyng, Francis, and Wenzel 2001).

Profit maximization in one's own part of the healthcare system has been and continues to be a common strategy. By itself this strategy leads to proliferation of underused competing facilities and collectively reduced profits as the investment cost of unneeded facilities is amortized. An alternative is to develop strategic relationships with partners representing the different parts of the healthcare system and maximize the collective profits for all.

The Future

Collaborative strategic partnerships and mutual trust are seen by many as required for future success (Anderson 2003; Mullins 2003; Reece 2003a, 2003b). The challenge for healthcare leaders is to look for ways to develop these strategic relationships that engage physicians and hospitals in each other's success. Steps in the process include:

1. seek to understand the needs of the other party first;
2. identify ways to help the other party meet its needs at the same time your needs are met;
3. look beyond what the other party will get to what you will get; and

4. remember that the objective is an agreement that works and endures—
   the financial benefit is not likely to be arithmetically equal.

It is a difficult process, but these steps are critical to developing collaborative strategic partnerships, building mutual trust, and engaging hospitals and physicians in each other's success.

Summary

Prior to the early 1990s physician and hospital services were seen as separate and distinct. The advancement of managed care as an economic force in healthcare and the early 1990s prospect of a national health plan requiring IDSs led to the conviction that hospitals needed to employ physicians to align hospitals and physicians in providing IDS care. With the failure of the Clinton health plan came a backlash against managed care. Payers turned to reducing fees paid rather than managed care as a way to control healthcare costs. Hospitals found that employed status did not produce the expected alignment with the employed physicians. What such status did produce was significant losses on the employed practices, and most hospitals divested them. Since the early 1990s advancing medical technology has blurred the lines between physician and hospital services. Declining reimbursement has provided a financial incentive for physicians to develop new services, often in competition with hospital services, to maintain and increase their incomes.

This chapter presents an overview of physician-hospital relationships, laws and regulations that proscribe those relationships, differing perspectives of physicians and hospital leadership that have inherent potential for conflict, and values held by most physicians and most hospital leaders. Many values are shared, and these provide the basis for developing collaborative strategic partnerships that well serve patients, physicians, hospitals, and communities. These collaborative partnerships build mutual trust and engage physicians and hospitals in each other's success.

Discussion Questions

1. Why did many hospitals decide in the early to mid-1990s that they
   needed to employ physicians? Why did many later decide to discontinue
   these employment arrangements?
2. What is causing hospitals and physicians to look again at ways of working
   more closely together?
3. How do joint ventures differ from other physician-hospital relationships?

4. Should lawyers be brought into the discussion of a possible joint venture as the first step in the discussion, or should they join it later? Why?
5. There is inherent conflict as the captain of the ship deals with the leader of the corporation. What steps can be taken to turn this conflict into a collaborative working relationship?
6. Why is it important to develop strategic relationships that engage physicians and hospitals in each other's success?

Notes

1. Most hospitals and health systems are not formally identified as corporations, but hospitals and health systems rival many corporations in their communities as the largest employer and organization with the highest revenue. Understandably many hospital and health system leaders see themselves as the equivalent of leaders of the corporation.
2. One example is the merger of two hospitals, with two different cultures, in a community. The hospital CEO set up a group with two nonsupervisory representatives from each hospital department—one from each of the two hospitals—and met with this group for a year, recording and distributing the questions raised and their answers. At the end of the year each member of the group was asked to pick his replacement to be in the group for the second year. This group continued in the following years, with the group serving the ongoing need for frequent meetings with employees.

References

Alexander, J. A., T. M. Waters, L. R. Burns, S. M. Shortell, R. R. Gillies, P. P. Budetti, and H. S. Zuckerman. 2001. "The Ties that Bind—Interorganizational Linkages and Physician-system Alignment." *Medical Care* 39 (7 Suppl. 1): 130–45.

Anderson, R. J. 2003. "Building Hospital-physician Relationships through Servant Leadership." *Frontiers of Health Services Management* 20 (2): 43–47.

Bujak, J. J. 2003. "How to Improve Hospital-physician Relationships." *Frontiers of Health Services Management* 20 (2): 3–21.

Flanakin, R. 2002. "The Conception, Demise and Resurrection of Physician Practice Management Companies." Fellowship Paper, American College of Medical Practice Executives. Englewood, CO: Medical Group Management Association.

Francis, D. M. 2004. Personal communication. Sept.

Jones, S. K. 2002. "Hospital/Physician Revenue Sharing Partnership." Fellowship Paper, American College of Medical Practice Executives. Englewood, CO: Medical Group Management Association.

Mitlyng, J. W., and F. J. Wenzel. 1999. "It Takes More than Money—Keys to Success in Leading and Managing Physician Groups." *Medical Group Management Journal* 46 (2): A30–38.

Mitlyng, J. W., D. M. Francis, and F. J. Wenzel. 2001. "Leaders as Combat Fighter Pilots." *The Physician Executive* 27 (6): 30–33.

Mullins, L. 2003. "Hospital-physician Relationships: A Synergy that Must Work." *Frontiers of Health Services Management* 20 (2): 37–41.

Reece, R. L. 2003a. "What Hospital CEOs Must Understand about the Physician Culture: Part 1." *HealthLeaders News* Oct. 3. [Online information.] www.healthleaders.com/news/feature1.php?contentid=48761.

———. 2003b. "What Hospital CEOs Must Understand about the Physician Culture: Part 2." *HealthLeaders News* Oct. 16. [Online information.] www.healthleaders.com/news/feature1.php?contentid=49271.

U.S. Department of Health and Human Services, Centers for Medicare & Medicaid Services. 2004. "Medicare Program; Physicians' Relationships with Health Care Entities with which they Have Financial Relationships (Phase II); Correction." *Federal Register* 69 (66): 17933–35.

U.S. Department of Justice. 1998. "Criminal Resource Manual 979 Health Care Fraud and Abuse Control Program" [Online information; retrieved 1/29/05.] www.usdoj.gov/usao/eousa/foia_reading_room/usam/title9/crm00979.htm.

THE FUTURE OF GROUP PRACTICE

Frederick J. Wenzel

Learning Objectives

This chapter will enable the reader to:

- place the future of group practice in perspective, considering both the past and present;
- understand the importance of physician organizations in a complex society and the role they will play in the future of the healthcare system;
- understand the drivers of the evolution of group practice, including values, quality, and cost;
- appreciate the role of group practice in the process of integration with other healthcare organizations (principally hospitals); and
- evaluate group practice as a career choice.

Chapter Purpose

This chapter provides a look at the future of group practice which is based on the dedication of the physicians, their contributions to the success of the professional organization, and the organization's ability to meet the needs of an ever-growing, complex healthcare system. Group practices are becoming more and more sophisticated, and they appear to be the model of choice for dealing with quality, disease, and demand management. Both single-specialty and multispecialty practices will continue to grow, and their leadership and management will become increasingly sophisticated. More and more physicians will seek training in leadership and management so they can effectively and efficiently deal with the complexity of their organizations. Quality will be the driver, and the tenets of the report *Crossing the Quality Chasm* will become the goals of healthcare organizations. Ownership of group practices by hospitals will decrease, and movement toward integration of the outpatient and inpatient environments will continue. Physicians will assume a stronger leadership role in healthcare systems through the group practice model, and students graduating from health administration programs will be attracted to working within such models.

Case in Point

Professor Allen was speaking to his students about careers in healthcare when one of the students asked about the potential of a management position in group practice and another student quickly responded with another question about the future of a group practice. Professor Allen thought for a moment and then began testing the knowledge of the students about the healthcare system which they had been studying for the past year. He framed their questions in light of relationships and the basic functions of the system which involve the physicians as the principal providers of direct medical care to the patients. He pointed out that it is the physicians who admit patients to the hospital and order tests and procedures to diagnose the patient's illness. He also pointed out that group practice has been growing very rapidly since the latter part of the last century, predicting that group practices would increase in numbers and grow ever larger because of the complexities in the system of the delivery of medical care services. He suggested that because of this growth and complexity there would be an increasing need for both physician and nonphysician managers and that the future of a group practice was bright. One of the students responded, "How can we learn more about group practice and its future?"

Impact of the Past and Present on the Future of Group Practice

It has been said that making predictions is difficult, especially when they are about the future. The same holds true about predicting the future of group practice. To begin the discussion the opinions of four professional consultants from the Medical Group Management Association (MGMA) were sought. Following are their thoughts.

Robert C. Bohlmann, FACMPE (2005)

In my opinion, a prognostication regarding the future of group practice must be based upon anticipated service needs, or market drivers, 5, 10, 15 years out. Patient service has always been a "given," but the manner in which service is provided has and will continue to change. Physician service has been and will continue to be in transition from a seller's to a buyer's market. The patient is now represented by employer, the government, unions, insurance carriers, and health plans. Quality, access, and the specter of cost escalation exceeding 16 to 17 percent of the gross domestic product all represent major concerns.

In order to successfully address stakeholder needs group practice will have to provide access and expand service hours, demonstrate quality, and exercise control over utilization. I anticipate the application of measurement tools, the capacity to manage resources, and the ability to work in a collaborative manner with patients and their representatives will be fundamental requirements of the successful group practice. If this needs assessment is correct, then group practices will tend to grow and adopt more characteristics of a formal service business. The consumer base will look to a single organization to provide comprehensive services; thus the multispecialty group, or one that can successfully subcontract for specialty services, will represent the optimum organizational format. The line between hospital and medical practice will continue to blur, with integrated systems regaining popularity (a trend now being observed). Capital needs will expand as technology and facility requirements grow. Thus outside investment may again bring Wall Street into the picture.

A major challenge will remain the balance between maintaining traditional medical services and adopting a more intense business orientation. Creation of a culture based upon physician ownership and comfort will be fundamental!

Darrell L. Schryver, DPA (2005)

The horizontal and vertical integration strategies of the 1990s were largely driven by market-based speculation. The primary motivation common among these models, whether in the form of a group practice merger, independent practice association (IPA), network, foundation models, or other forms of a vertically integrated delivery system (IDS), was largely based on the presumption that size provides greater market opportunities. More precisely, a network was required to gain access to managed care contracts and have greater control over the price of those contracts to enhance the integrated venture's market position. It is my opinion the IDS will evolve/reemerge over the next 25 years into the primary vehicle for the delivery of health services in a significant number of communities nationally. Upon closer review the IDS model will provide an opportunity for physicians and hospitals, as the primary components of the healthcare delivery system, to plan together strategically in order to: (1) ensure the future viability of a community's healthcare delivery system; and (2) provide the community with appropriate quality and efficient healthcare services. These goals reflect the changing healthcare system. With the trends of increased costs and declining reimbursement, the goal(s) related to the integrated delivery system will shift from market control to assuring the future long-term viability of a community's delivery system and the provision of essential physician and other healthcare services to the community at large.

Hobart Collins, CMPE (2005)

The future of medical groups is bright; the only constant will be change. In terms of numbers the vast majority of physicians will be members of medical groups. The actual number of medical groups may increase or decrease depending on local market factors and consolidation trends/results.

Single-specialty groups, at least in the more highly remunerated specialties, will continue to grow for obvious self-serving reasons. There may be a trend to increasing numbers of multidisciplinary groups organized around narrow systems or diseases, for example, neurosciences (neurology, interventional neuroradiology, and neurosurgery), cardiovascular services (cardiology, interventional radiology, CT surgery), and others.

The future of large and all-encompassing multispecialty groups is less clear. Existing groups will continue to expand; it is likely the number of megagroups will not expand significantly.

There will be another round of "physician practice management" companies, this time perhaps with some success. This will occur primarily because physicians are attracted to seeking a higher position in the food chain. There will also be another round of "managed care," at least in suitable markets or regions.

If total healthcare expenditures begin to approach 20 percent of the GDP, the pressures for a reasonable all-payer system will be enormous. A collaborative model (involving patients, providers, and payers) will become a reality as the only sensible public policy approach capable of a long-term "solution."

Other areas of focus likely are:

1. Accountability: evidence-based medicine will be the gold standard, with uniform protocols in place broadly if not universally.
2. Technology will continue to challenge geographic boundaries as certain specialties such as radiology are able to operate on a global basis.
3. Ownership will continue to evolve; there will be large numbers of public-private partnerships.

Richard D. Hansen, MS (2005)

In the next ten years medical groups will combine cultural and technological integration to ensure the most customer-oriented and efficient delivery systems possible. Mission and vision will be clearly communicated and will empower everyone in the practice to do their best. Always aware that practices, like all human organizations, serve and are served by human beings, mistakes will be made, but the most successful groups will use those "bumps in the road" to design even better delivery systems.

Comments

A number of issues emerge from the comments made by these MGMA consultants, including access, cost, quality, automation, and integration.

Access means two things, the first of which is providing patients with an opportunity to be seen at the most appropriate time. The second factor is equity in access, which means that all individuals will have an equal opportunity to be seen regardless of gender, race, or ability to pay. The U.S. healthcare system is a long way from solving these problems, but discussions at the professional, community, and governmental levels appear headed in the right direction.

Cost looms over the healthcare system with little hope for a solution in the near term. Many things have been attempted, such as differing reimbursement systems, managed care, cuts in the Medicare and Medicaid programs, and so forth, to little avail. The search for answers continues.

The publication of *Crossing the Quality Chasm* and *To Err Is Human* significantly increased the attention paid at all levels to the quality and safety of healthcare services. A number of physician organizations are leading the studies in this area, sponsored by the Center for Medicare and Medicaid Services. These studies are being augmented by further work on pay-for-performance systems, in which physicians and institutions are being reimbursed on the basis of quality and adherence to certain standards. At this point the jury is out.

Some of the predictions of the consultants involved technological expansion. There is no doubt that automation, especially the electronic medical record, will be one of the drivers of the future.

It was suggested that group practices should balance their service and business orientation and create a culture based on physician ownership and comfort. Also of interest is the prediction about the reemergence of the IDS on a national basis. If physicians and hospitals can plan together as they envision the future, the opportunity for developing a system that delivers effective and efficient care would be much greater than if the organizations proceeded on their separate paths. The IDSs would shift from market control to service orientation under physician leadership.

The experts consulted expressed a significant degree of optimism and even suggested that practice management firms would again emerge along with the resurgence of managed care. The principal factors involved in this process are quality, cost, accountability, technology, and public-private partnerships. These factors, when added together, appear to herald a new growth phase for group practices over the next 10 to 25 years.

The consultants voiced a number of interesting opinions on the growth of group practice, and while all seem to agree it will continue, that growth may take different forms. Collins (2005) pointed out that most of the growth will be in single-specialty and multidisciplinary organizations. While the numbers of physicians in large multispecialty practices will grow, the number of large group practices will likely remain about the same.

Drivers of the Future of Group Practice

The drivers of the future of group practice have been well-defined by the consultants and are embedded or implied in the following trends:

- Patient and payer insistence on high quality and its evaluation
- System control over costs
- The move toward pay-for-performance initiatives
- The government stressing technological advancements, especially in information systems
- Resurgence of interest in integrated systems by physicians and hospitals
- Increasing complexity from every aspect of healthcare delivery and its regulation
- Strengthening physician leadership

It appears that there has been a temporary, modest rise in healthcare spending, which will ease the pressure for radical reform. However, there is no doubt that the trends listed above will continue to drive change in the healthcare system. Much of this change will be reflected in group practices. Physicians drive the economic engine by admitting patients to hospitals and ordering complex tests and treatments; this will become more of an influence in the years to come.

Complex Healthcare Systems

At one time the conventional wisdom was that the IDS would be the answer to the development of effectiveness and efficiency in the delivery of healthcare services. That process began in earnest in the late 1980s and proceeded into the 1990s. Many hospitals purchased group practices only to find that they were unable to manage the professionals and the cost of having physician groups integrated into the system was too high to continue. Therefore, a significant move toward divestiture and system disintegration occurred in the late 1990s and on into this century.

It may well be that while a resurgence in the development of integrated systems will occur, it will not be because of the economics of the hospital or the need for the physician groups to have a home; rather development will be driven by the complexity of the system itself. Logic dictates that a time will come when both physicians and hospitals conclude that the best way to deliver healthcare services is through an integrated system led by professionals with a continuum of care from the ambulatory clinic to the hospital if necessary and back again to ambulatory care. In this system great attention will be paid to prevention and health maintenance. The delivery of healthcare services has become an extremely complex process, and it is only rational that this delivery system can best be housed in a complex, integrated healthcare organization.

The Quality Imperative

The demand for quality will continue, and quality evaluation can best be performed under an organizational umbrella including both the hospital and group practice setting. The advantage of evaluating quality in an integrated system is that the process involves the entire continuum of care, not just one aspect or phase. If the system is to move beyond process and into outcomes, it is reasonable to conclude that all factors involved in patient care should be evaluated as part of the outcome model.

As the value equation is represented by quality/cost, it is not difficult to see that when quality increases even though costs remain the same, the value represented in the equation rises sharply. This is a most difficult task and cannot be accomplished without the full cooperation of physicians, especially those in group practices. To ignore this aspect of the quality imperative is to bury one's head in the sand.

At the same time a great deal of attention must be paid to quality in the eyes of the patient, which of course often has little resemblance to quality in the eyes of the professional. Although patients are always interested in getting well, they are also interested in getting an appointment at the appropriate time, being seen promptly, the physician taking time with them and answering their questions, and being treated with dignity. Quality from the prospective of both the professional and patient must be considered.

Information Systems and Information Technology

The surface has barely been scratched in information systems and technology. Automating business systems has led the way, followed now by automation of patient information systems from appointment systems to ordering tests, reporting, prescribing, and medical records. These innovations will lead the way to advances in patient care that were previously not thought possible.

The next step will be linking systems throughout the country. This began in earnest in 2004, when President Bush created the Office for National Health Information Technology and David Brailer, M.D., Ph.D., was appointed its director. Dr. Brailer's vision is to create a national health information network with a standard scheme for information transfer and information technology network organization; included is a federal commitment to coordinating the use of specific standards and computer applications throughout government agencies that deal with healthcare delivery. The new organization will not only be responsible for interorganizational information transfer but will also be a vehicle for broad-based clinical and business applications, including disease management programs and pay-for-performance initiatives. Group practices, especially large multispecialty groups, are poised to participate in these developments.

Future Growth of Organizational Models

Single-Specialty Groups

These groups will continue to grow in numbers as well as size. Mergers among single-specialty groups may be constrained by antitrust laws. Some of these groups will become more like multispecialty clinics, adding additional specialties to support their service delivery. It is not unusual for a group of family physicians to discover that having pediatricians or surgeons in their group makes referrals easier and offers convenience to their patients.

Multispecialty Groups

These groups will not grow in number, but their size will increase significantly. The greatest number of physicians will be found in these clinics. They will also form the backbone of large IDSs.

Academic Health Centers

Medical schools that previously had departmental practice plans will form group practice foundations in which the physicians will be housed in a single organization. They will emulate the large multispecialty groups and absorb some of the primary care and specialty groups located in their communities.

Systems and Hospital Groups

The current large delivery systems composed of hospitals and physician groups will for the most part survive. There will be a continuing move toward systems with group practices rather than hospitals as the nucleus (i.e., The Mayo Model).

Leadership and Mangement of the Future

As the healthcare system becomes more physician driven there will be a significant need for physician leaders and managers. Although these individuals must first and foremost have outstanding clinical credentials, there will be a continuing need for them to obtain academic credentials in business leadership and management. The ideal healthcare system will be led and managed by a team of physicians and nonphysicians at all levels of the organization.

A number of different models are evolving around the country; they will be tested for their ability to survive and thrive over the next five to ten years. These models include the Mayo System, Cleveland Clinic, MeritCare in Fargo, North Dakota, Virginia Mason in Seattle, Geisinger Health System in Danville, Pennsylvania, Scott & White in Temple, Texas, and others. The need for managers at all levels of the organization will be significant and provide opportunity for students from healthcare management programs at the undergraduate and graduate levels. The competencies for these staff members have been described in detail by Ross, Mitlyng, and Wenzel (2002) in *Leadership for the Future*.

Summary—Where Will It All End?

That is the question! We might begin by quoting Herzlinger (1999), when she predicted who would be rewarded in the new healthcare system: "It will be those who deliver what the marketing message promises, those with comprehensive clinical and managerial control systems and those whose managerial philosophy focuses on the organizational purpose." It will all end with insistence on high quality, high tech with high touch, genetic engineering, spare-parts technology, focus on the chronic diseases of aging, emphasis on the impact of behavioral factors, and ultimately a changed healthcare system. Group practice will play a major role in all of these areas.

Discussion Questions

1. Where are group practices headed as an organizational model?
2. Should physicians take responsibility and be accountable for the delivery system?
3. Why does integration seem to be a future trend?
4. What are the advantages of large multispecialty clinics?
5. What will the role of the hospital be in these developments?
6. How can physicians prepare themselves for the role of responsibility and accountability?

References

Bohlmann, R. C. 2005. Personal communication. Jan. 12.

Collins, H. 2005. Personal communication. Jan. 17.

Hansen, R. D. 2005. Personal communication. Jan. 20.

Herzlinger, R. 1999. *Market-driven Health Care: Who Wins, Who Loses in the Transformation of America's Largest Service Industry*. New York: Perseus.

Ross, A., J. W. Mitlyng, and F. J. Wenzel. 2002. *Leadership for the Future: Core Competencies in Healthcare*. Chicago: Health Administration Press.

Schryver, D. L. 2005. Personal communication. Jan. 15.

SUGGESTED READING LIST

Andreasen, A. R. 1995. *Marketing Social Change*. San Francisco: Jossey-Bass.

Baker, J. J., and R. W. Baker. 2000. *Health Care Finance: Basic Tools for Non-financial Managers*. Gaithersburg, MD: Aspen Publishers.

Barton, P. L. 2003. *Understanding the U.S. Health Services System, Second Edition*. Chicago: Health Administration Press.

Berkowitz, E. N. 2004. *Essentials of Healthcare Marketing*. Boston: Jones and Bartlett.

Clemmer, J. 1992. *Firing on All Cylinders—Service/Quality for High Powered Corporate Performance*. Homewood, IL: Business One Irwin.

Coddington, D. C., K. D. Moore, and R. L. Clarke. 1998. *Capitalizing Medical Groups: Positioning Physicians for the Future*. New York: McGraw-Hill.

Coile, R. C. 1997. *The Five Stages of Managed Care: Strategies for Providers, HMOs, and Suppliers*. Chicago: Health Administration Press.

Collins, J. C., and J. I. Porras. 1994. *Built to Last: Successful Habits of Visionary Companies*. New York: HarperBusiness.

Dawes, R. M. 1988. *Rational Choice in an Uncertain World*. Orlando, FL: Harcourt Brace Jovanovich.

Deal, T. E., and A. A. Kennedy. 1982. *Corporate Cultures: The Rites and Rituals of Corporate Life*. Boston: Addison-Wesley.

de Geus, A. 1997. *The Living Company*. Boston: Harvard Business School Press.

Drucker, P., P. Senge, and F. Hesselbein. 2001. *Leading in a Time of Change*. San Francisco: Jossey-Bass.

Fortenberry, J. L. 2005. *Marketing Tools for Healthcare Executives*. Oxford, MI: Oxford Crest.

Fottler, M., R. C. Ford, and C. P. Heaton. 2002. *Achieving Service Excellence: Strategies for Healthcare*. Chicago: Health Administration Press.

Gapenski, L. C. 2004. *Healthcare Finance: An Introduction to Accounting and Financial Management, Third Edition*. Chicago: Health Administration Press.

Getzen, T. E. 2004. *Health Economics—Fundamental and Flow of Funds*. New York: John Wiley & Sons, Inc.

Griffith, J. R., and K. R. White. 2002. *The Well-Managed Healthcare Organization*, 5th ed. Chicago: Health Administration Press.

Harris, D. M. 2003. *Contemporary Issues in Healthcare, Law and Ethics*, 2nd ed. Chicago: Health Administration Press.

Hekman, K. M. 1997. *Buying, Selling & Merging a Medical Practice*. Englewood, CO: Medical Group Management Association.

Herzlinger, R. E. 1997. *Market-Driven Health Care: Who Wins, Who Loses in the Transformation of America's Largest Service Industry*. New York: Perseus Books.

Hesselbein, F., M. Goldsmith, and R. Beckhard (eds.). 1996. *The Leader of the Future*. San Franciso: Jossey-Bass.

Hillestead, S. G., and E. N. Berkowitz. 2003. *Healthcare Market Strategy*. Boston: Jones and Bartlett.

Kotler, P. 2003. *Marketing Management*. Upper Saddle River, NJ: Prentice Hall.

Luke, R. D., S. L. Walston, and P. M. Plummer. 2004. *Healthcare Strategy: In Pursuit of Competitive Advantage*. Chicago: Health Administration Press.

Nowicki, M. 2004. *The Financial Management of Hospitals and Healthcare Organizations, Third Edition*. Chicago: Health Administration Press.

Pattee, J. J., and O. J. Otteson. 1997. *The Health Care Future: Defining the Argument, Healing the Debate*. Plymouth, MN: North Ridge Press.

Pointer, D. D., and J. E. Orlikoff. 1999. *Board Work*. San Francisco: Jossey-Bass.

Pozgar, G. 2004. *Legal Aspects of Health Care Administration*. Boston: Jones and Bartlett.

Ransom, S. B., M. Joshi and D. B. Nash, (eds.). 2004. *The Healthcare Quality Book: Vision, Strategy and Tools*. Chicago: Health Administration Press.

Ross, A., S. J. Williams, and E. J. Pavlock. 1998. *Ambulatory Care Management*. Albany, NY: Delmar Publishers, Inc.

Rubin, I. M. 1991. *My Pulse Is Not What it Used to Be*. Honolulu: The Temenos Foundation.

Senge, P. 1994. *The Fifth Discipline: The Art and Practice of the Learning Organization*. New York: Currency/Doubleday.

Shortell, S. M., R. G. Gillies, D. A. Anderson, K. M. Erickson, and J. B. Mitchell. 2000. *Remaking Health Care in America*. San Francisco: Jossey-Bass.

Showalter, J. S. 2004. *The Law of Healthcare Administration, Fourth Edition*. Chicago: Health Administration Press.

Turner, C. H. 1992. *Creating Corporate Culture*. Boston: Addison-Wesley.

Williams, C. A., M. L. Smith, and P. C. Young. 1998. *Risk Management and Insurance*. Boston: Irwin McGraw-Hill.

INDEX

ABOUT THE CONTRIBUTORS

Frederick J. Wenzel, M.B.A., FACMPE

Frederick J. Wenzel, MBA, FACMPE, is professor and academic director of the MBA program in Medical Group Management at the College of Business at the University of St. Thomas. He also holds a visiting appointment with the Graduate School of Business at the University of Colorado. He is a graduate of the University of Wisconsin and the Graduate School of Business of the University of Chicago.

Mr. Wenzel served as executive director of the Marshfield Clinic Research and Education Foundation for 16 years, then as executive director of the Marshfield Clinic for 17 years. He now serves on the clinic's National Advisory Council and is advisor to the president of the clinic. He was executive vice president and CEO of the Medical Group Management Association (MGMA) and the American College of Medical Practice Executives (ACMPE) from 1993 to 1996. He served on the Accreditation Commission for Education in Health Service Administration, where he completed two years as chair of the Commission. Mr. Wenzel also serves on the boards of Marshall Erdman and Associates, University of Wisconsin Medical Foundation, Health Quality Partners, Fairview Physician Associates, and American Cancer Society, Midwest Division.

In addition to writing and teaching Mr. Wenzel speaks at regional and national conferences and consults with healthcare organizations throughout the country. With his colleagues Austin Ross and Joseph Mitlyng, he has published a book on the future of healthcare leadership competencies. He holds a master's degree of business administration from the University of Chicago and is a fellow of ACMPE.

Jane M. Wenzel, Ph.D.

Jane Wenzel, Ph.D., has combined experience in the academic environment with her expertise in organization and design to provide services as an instructional designer in the development of virtual classrooms on the Internet. Jane works closely with faculty in the translation of syllabi and course content using the distance learning model to develop Internet-based virtual classrooms. In addition to course design and input, she provides instruction to faculty and students as well as technical support. Jane also works with professional groups and organizations in using this same technology for improving communication and providing continuing professional education.

Jane began her own successful desktop publishing business ten years ago providing services to professional organizations, healthcare organizations (non-profit), consultants, and small business owners in southern Wisconsin. She provides direct service and consultation in the organization, development, and production of annual reports, employee and board member handbooks, forms, calendars, educational materials and marketing materials such as newsletters and brochures. Other services Jane provides are technical and grant proposal writing, database management, computer technical support, software/hardware purchase, installation and maintenance.

Jane received her doctorate from the University of Wisconsin–Madison and has been published in a number of peer-reviewed professional journals. Jane and Fritz have worked together for the last ten years. Fritz shares Jane's enthusiasm for online learning and they have made numerous presentations together on the subject. Jane also assists Fritz in all aspects of his teaching, consulting, and work as a writer.

Rosemarie Nelson, M.S.

Rosemarie Nelson, M.S., is a senior consultant with the MGMA HealthCare Consulting Group. Her experience in information technology and as a medical office manager, combined with her years of consulting to physicians and practice professionals, gives her a unique insight into the needs and challenges facing today's physicians and the future for medical practices. Ms. Nelson conducts educational seminars and provides keynote speeches on a variety of healthcare technology and operational topics. She has authored numerous articles on practice management issues, and her seminar presentations and publications have been well-received by physicians, administrators, office managers, and staff throughout the country.

As a medical practice consultant Rosemarie has established significant expertise in system implementation. As a manager in the multimanufacturer Office of the Future project, she led new technology planning and development for improved clinical operations. She has managed project implementation teams as well as software engineers in design, implementation, and training for medical practice software.

Ms. Nelson serves on the boards of the American Heart Association North East Affiliate and the Syracuse University Orange Pack. She was awarded the 2000 Professional Achievement Award by New School University, Robert J. Milano Graduate School of Management & Urban Policy. Ms. Nelson serves as faculty in Health IT Certification and adjunct faculty at the University of St. Thomas, teaching in the MBA in Medical Group Management program.

Ms. Nelson has a master of science degree in health services administration from The New School for Social Research Graduate School of Management and Urban Policy and a bachelor of science degree in management of information systems from Syracuse University.

Joseph W. Mitlyng, M.B.A., FACMPE

Joseph W. Mitlyng, M.B.A., FACMPE, is president of Mitlyng Associates, Inc., a healthcare management consulting firm he founded in 1994. The mission of Mitlyng Associates is:

> Developing Strategic Relationships
> that Engage Physicians and Hospitals
> in Each Other's Success

Clients have included hospitals, health systems, academic medical centers, and physician groups. Consulting services have included the areas of governance, leadership, and management of physician groups and physician-hospital organizations; operations improvement; and compensation. Mr. Mitlyng has also served as an interim executive with hands-on line management responsibility for financial turnarounds.

Mr. Mitlyng was executive vice president and COO of Park Nicollet Medical Center from 1986 to 1994, during a major turnaround period. Before taking his position at Park Nicollet, he was associate director of the Marshfield Clinic from 1975 to 1986. In 1994 he was president of MGMA.

He is the lead author of "It Takes More than Money—Keys to Success in Leading and Managing Physician Groups" and "Leaders as Combat Fighter Pilots," and he is a coauthor of *Leadership for the Future: Core Competencies in Healthcare* (Health Administration Press 2001). He is featured in *Trials to Triumphs: Perspectives of Successful Healthcare Leaders* (Health Administration Press 2001).

Mr. Mitlyng has a master's degree in business from Harvard Business School and is a fellow of ACMPE.

Joseph P. White, C.P.A., M.B.A.

Joseph P. White, C.P.A., M.B.A., is a principal at Larson Allen Weishair & Co., LLP, a national accounting and consulting firm in Minneapolis. He is adjunct faculty at the University of St. Thomas, teaching in the MBA in Medical Group Management program, Center for Health and Medical Affairs, Physician Leadership College, and Mini-MBA in Medical Group Management program. He also teaches graduate-level finance courses at Argosy University.

Mr. White graduated from the University of Minnesota with a bachelor's degree with an emphasis in accounting and received an MBA from the University of St. Thomas. He is a licensed CPA and a member of MGMA,

Minnesota Medical Group Management Association, American Institute of Certified Public Accountants, Minnesota Society of Certified Public Accountants, and Health Care Financial Management Association. Joe has been named a "Super CPA" by *Twin Cities Business Monthly* and *Minnesota Law & Politics* several times.

Mr. White's expertise is in working with physician groups and other healthcare organizations. He focuses largely on strategic planning and positioning of healthcare organizations and healthcare mergers, acquisitions, and affiliations. Mr. White is actively involved in financial and operations improvement; the typical context for most of his engagements is that of helping organizations find strategic, financial, and operational solutions for their businesses. Mr. White's clients include large and small single-specialty and multispecialty physician practice organizations, large community healthcare systems, and rural healthcare providers.

Mr. White has a broad foundation of technical expertise within the healthcare arena. He leads physician practice consulting for Larson Allen and has experience in tax, accounting, finance, reimbursement, and operational issues. He has authored numerous articles related to tax, finance, and accounting topics and speaks frequently on issues related to physician organizations.